ATLAS OF
STRABISMUS SURGERY

ATLAS OF
STRABISMUS SURGERY

Eugene M. Helveston, M.D.

Professor of Ophthalmology,
Indiana University School of Medicine,
Indianapolis, Indiana

SECOND EDITION

with 382 illustrations in 97 plates

The C. V. Mosby Company

Saint Louis   1977

SECOND EDITION

Copyright © 1977 by The C. V. Mosby Company

All rights reserved. No part of this book may be reproduced
in any manner without written permission of the publisher.

Previous edition copyrighted 1973

Printed in the United States of America

Distributed in Great Britain by Henry Kimpton, London

The C. V. Mosby Company
11830 Westline Industrial Drive, St. Louis, Missouri 63141

Library of Congress Cataloging in Publication Data

Helveston, Eugene M   1934-
    Atlas of strabismus surgery.

    Bibliography: p.
    Includes index.
    1. Strabismus—Surgery—Atlases.   I. Title.
[DNLM: 1. Strabismus—Surgery—Atlases.
WW17 H485a]
RE771.H4   1977   617.7′62   77-3542
ISBN 0-8016-2138-0

TS/U/B   9   8   7   6   5   4   3   2   1

With love and gratitude
to my wife
BARBARA

Foreword

The principles of strabismus surgery, consisting of weakening the action of an overacting muscle or strengthening the action of an underacting muscle, have remained unchanged for many years. Significant modifications and refinements during the last few decades, however, have enabled the surgeon to deal more effectively with clinical situations in strabismus, many of which were thought to be incurable only a short time ago. For instance, the improved preoperative and intraoperative diagnosis of mechanical factors and their elimination by conjunctival surgery and other means, the increased popularity and proved effectiveness of muscle transposition procedures, the use of plastic materials, the improvement of exposure techniques for surgery on the oblique muscles, and the reintroduction of marginal myotomies are some of the features that have recently received special attention.

Descriptions of these and other modern surgical approaches are scattered widely in the literature and are not readily accessible to most ophthalmologists. This atlas fills a definite void in presenting an up-to-date collection of current surgical techniques and indications for their use.

Dr. Helveston, an experienced strabismus surgeon, is a well-qualified authority on the subject. He has performed an invaluable service in assembling this atlas. The wealth of illustrative material and the accompanying succinct text should make this book indispensable for residents and ophthalmologists in practice. I predict that it will be received enthusiastically by the ophthalmologic community and am proud that it comes from the pen of one of my former students.

Gunter K. von Noorden

Professor of Ophthalmology,
Baylor College of Medicine,
Houston, Texas

Preface TO SECOND EDITION

In the 4 years since publication of the first edition, several new surgical techniques have become popularized, some older techniques have been refined, improved suture materials have been developed, and testing procedures have advanced in the field of ophthalmology. The Faden operation, or posterior fixation suture, has found a variety of uses. A simplified adjustable suture has proved extremely useful in the management of strabismus with restriction, as has expanded use of conjunctival recession. Synthetic absorbable sutures, while not yet of the ideal design, are probably made of the ideal material for buried sutures where absorption is desirable. Force and velocity tests have found expanded use.

Increased surgical volume and greater follow-up time produces widened experience, and this prompted several minor changes in the text. The occurrence of more and unique complications was expected; these will also be included.

Much of the material for this edition was obtained with the assistance and criticism of my colleague, Dr. Forrest D. Ellis. As in the first edition, Craig G. Gosling provided the illustrations.

The many readers of the first edition, including residents, fellows, and fellow ophthalmologists, supported my efforts by acknowledging what they thought was worthwhile and by offering suggestions for changes and additions where they thought such modification would be beneficial. Many thanks also to Joanna Jackson for typing the manuscript.

Eugene M. Helveston

Preface TO FIRST EDITION

There have been several excellent texts on strabismus including strabismus surgery in the past few years, but developments have moved rapidly. Recent advances in technique have greatly expanded the options available to the strabismus surgeon. More accurate diagnostic tests leading to a better understanding of the pathophysiology of strabismus and amblyopia have convinced some surgeons of the need for surgery in infants as young as 5 months of age. Improved anesthesia and an increasing boldness on the part of the strabismus surgeon have led to outpatient extraocular muscle surgery in some instances without patch and without ointment or drops. The limbal and cul-de-sac (or fornix) extraocular muscle exposure techniques have largely superseded the transconjunctival incision in the interpalpebral space among younger surgeons. The retinal surgeon has opened new dimensions in the degree to which sub-Tenon's space may be explored.

New sutures, adhesives, muscle sleeves, and implantation materials have proved useful innovations. Globe fixation sutures, conjunctival recession and relaxation procedures, forced duction and active forced generation tests, as well as topical anesthesia for extraocular muscle surgery, have greatly enlarged the vista of strabismus surgery.

For these reasons it seems appropriate at this time to compile an up-to-date atlas of strabismus surgery. This atlas employs schematic drawings designed to illustrate at each step only that anatomy significant to the step shown for easier orientation of the reader. Procedures that I have found useful have been given emphasis; those that are controversial or that I have not found to be particularly helpful have been omitted. A "favorite technique" may be omitted simply because I prefer an alternative choice; those that I think should be avoided will be clearly labeled so.

No attempt will be made to give a set of surgical recipes that will result in a predetermined amount of straightening. Instead, general concepts leading to a philosophy for strabismus surgery will be presented. My intent is that this atlas will be of help to the practicing strabismus surgeon and the resident in ophthalmology by bringing together in one volume many techniques from a variety of sources for quick and easy reference.

Several people who assisted significantly in their own way to make this atlas possible deserve my sincere thanks. Dr. Gunter K. von Noorden, teacher, critic, and friend, introduced me to strabismus and to the pursuit of academic ophthalmology. Craig G. Gosling worked with industry and imagination on the illustrations, the heart of any atlas. Ken Julian, Susan Argeroplos, and Joe Demma prepared the photographic material. Dr. Fred M. Wilson provided the departmental leadership that made it possible to complete this work. Dr. Merrill Grayson furnished helpful criticism. Bonnie Wilson made the operating room a pleasant place in which to work. My residents and many of my colleagues, in particular Drs. Marshall M. Parks and Phillip Knapp, provided both stimulus and direction. My thanks also to Mrs. Paul Sanders and Pamela L. Payne for typing the manuscript.

Eugene M. Helveston

Contents

ATLAS OF
STRABISMUS SURGERY

CHAPTER ONE

Surgical anatomy

A clear understanding of the anatomy of the extraocular muscles and of the fascial structures associated with the globe and orbit is a prerequisite to successful strabismus surgery. The conjunctiva, anterior Tenon's capsule, posterior Tenon's capsule (intermuscular membrane), and muscle sheath play an important part in the movement of the globe. These structures perform a passive role in ocular movement with regard to initiation of movement, but they play an active role with regard to restriction of movement. Proper management of these structures can often spell the difference between successful and unsuccessful strabismus surgery.

The surgeon must be concerned with the mechanics of access to the operative site between the lids and through the conjunctiva and Tenon's capsule. A proper beginning is an obvious requisite to a successful conclusion. The location as well as the blood supply, innervation, and action of each extraocular muscle must be known, including the contribution of each muscle's intrinsic blood supply to the nutrition of the anterior segment of the globe. The scleral thickness, which varies according to location, must be taken into account when choosing needles to place into the sclera.

THE PALPEBRAL FISSURE

The dimensions of the palpebral opening increase nearly 50% in width and 20% in height between infancy and adulthood. The configuration of the palpebral opening varies with a person's physical and racial characteristics.

PLATE 1-1

A   The average adult palpebral opening is 28 mm long and 10 mm high. A solid blade, spring-loaded lid speculum with 18-mm blades effectively holds the lids widely apart to provide ample exposure for extraocular muscle surgery. In performing extraocular muscle surgery, the lids are separated without concern for a slightly increased intraocular pressure; with intraocular surgery, however, increased intraocular pressure *is* a great concern.

B   The average 18-month-old child has a palpebral opening that is 20 mm long and 8.5 mm high. A solid blade lid speculum with 8-mm blades is adequate for most children of this age.

C   The newborn has a palpebral opening measuring 18 mm long and 8 mm high. A solid blade lid speculum with 6-mm blades is adequate for the newborn.

The size of the palpebral opening is a significant factor in extraocular muscle surgery technique. A lid speculum appropriate to the size of the palpebral opening should be used. The surgeon should also expect to encounter more difficulty with exposure and suture placement, particularly in medial rectus recession, in patients with a small palpebral fissure or deeply set eyes. However, measured recession can be accomplished even with the smallest lid fissure opening in a 6-month-old child. Limited working area is not an adequate reason for doing a marginal myotomy as an initial weakening procedure of a medial rectus muscle in infantile esotropia, simply because the marginal myotomy is easier to accomplish than a measured recession. Extraocular surgery in an adult with deeply set eyes and a smaller than average palpebral opening can be more difficult than such surgery in a 3- or 4-year-old child with a normal or larger than normal palpebral opening.

Unlike the palpebral opening, which is a significantly different size in adults, infants, and young children, the extraocular muscles are nearly equal in size throughout life. A child with a tiny palpebral opening is likely to have a medial rectus whose insertion is very close to the adult measurements of approximately 10 mm wide. The timing of early surgery is not in any way limited by the size of the palpebral opening or of the extraocular muscles.

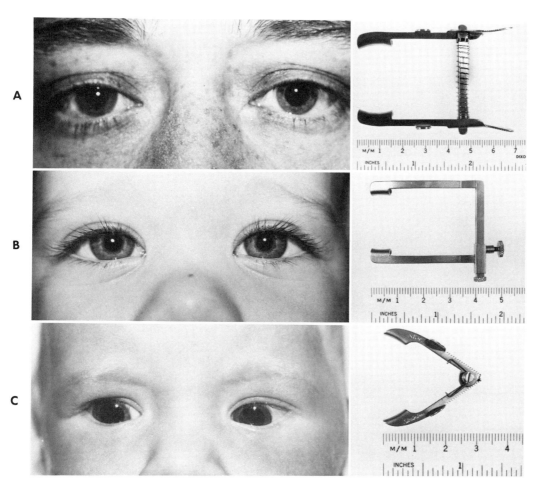

PLATE 1-1

The palpebral fissure may be level, mongoloid, or antimongoloid, depending on the relative positions of the medial and lateral canthi. If the outer canthus is higher than the inner canthus, a mongoloid palpebral slant exists. If the outer canthus is lower than the inner canthus, an antimongoloid palpebral slant exists. A straightedge held in front of the palpebral fissure connecting the canthi may be used to compare the relative canthal height. The "normal" relative canthal height is dependent upon what is considered normal for a given race. In whites, the palpebral fissure is usually slightly "mongoloid"—that is, the lateral canthus is slightly higher than the medial canthus. Careful measurements of the Oriental palpebral fissure indicate less mongoloid slant than would be expected from casual observation. The mongoloid illusion in many cases is accentuated by the lack of a skin fold in the upper lid.

The palpebral fissure configuration imparts a characteristic appearance to an individual including, at times, a pseudostrabismus. Vertically incomitant strabismus (A and V patterns) in esotropia follow a pattern related to the slant of the fissures. This was first pointed out by Urrets-Zavalia. In esotropia, a mongoloid fissure is associated with an A pattern, an antimongoloid fissure with a V pattern. No firm anatomic basis for this relationship has been established. In exodeviations there seems to be no such correlation. When examining a strabismus patient who has either a mongoloid or an antimongoloid lid fissure, one should always be on the lookout for vertical incomitance.

PLATE 1-2

A V esotropia in a patient with antimongoloid palpebral fissures.
B A esotropia in a patient with mongoloid palpebral fissures.

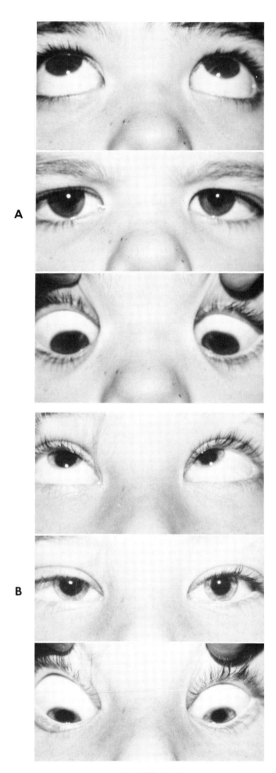

A

B

PLATE 1-2

Epicanthal folds are present to some degree in most children during the first few years of life. These skin folds create an illusion of esotropia, and many children are referred to the ophthalmologist because of this pseudoesotropia. Parents think one eye turns in because no "white" can be seen medially, especially in the adducted eye in lateral versions. Two techniques can be employed to relieve the parents' concern regarding the pseudoesotropia of epicanthus. These are (1) to demonstrate the centered pupillary reflexes with a muscle light and (2) to pull the skin forward over the bridge of the nose, demonstrating the "straightening" effect of exposing medial conjunctiva. It is still a good rule for the ophthalmologist confronted with an obvious case of pseudostrabismus to perform a complete eye examination, including cycloplegic refraction and retinal examination. A portable, indirect ophthalmoscope is invaluable for infant retinal examination in such cases.

PLATE 1-3

A Epicanthal folds obscure the nasal conjunctiva in both patients, giving the appearance of esotropia. However, the light reflex is centered in the pupil in each case. This indicates the presence of parallel pupillary axes and therefore straight eyes or absence of manifest strabismus. Cover testing must be done eventually to confirm the presence of parallel visual axes because a large angle kappa* could hide a small manifest deviation.

B Epicanthal folds are present, but the displaced pupillary reflex in the right eye confirms the presence of a right esotropia.

C A skin fold originating below and sweeping upward is called epicanthus inversus. This deformity is frequently associated with blepharophimosis and ptosis. This triad of deformities causes a significant disfigurement and presents a formidable therapeutic challenge.

---

*Angle kappa is the angle formed by the pupillary axis and the visual axis. A positive angle kappa is present when the visual axis is nasal to the pupillary axis. This simulates exotropia and is common. A negative angle kappa is present when the visual axis is temporal to the pupillary axis. This simulates esotropia, and it is much less common than positive angle kappa.

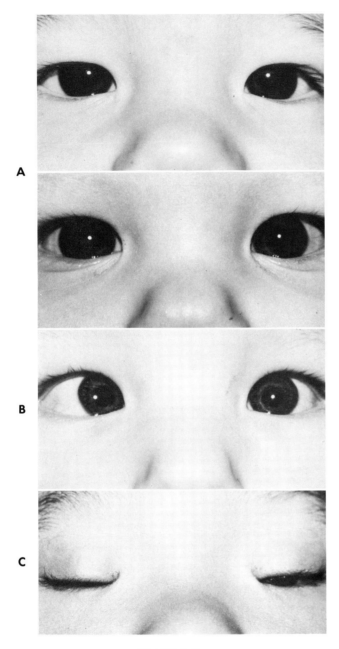

A

B

C

PLATE 1-3

THE CONJUNCTIVA

The bulbar conjunctiva loosely covers the anterior part of the globe from the fornices above and below and from the canthi medially and laterally. It becomes fused with anterior Tenon's capsule and the sclera at the limbus. The conjunctiva is thick and has substance in infancy and childhood, but it becomes much thinner and more friable in adulthood and senility.

PLATE 1-4

Landmarks of the conjunctiva important to the strabismus surgeon are:
- A 1 The fusion of conjunctiva and anterior Tenon's capsule with sclera at the limbus
  - 2 The plica semilunaris
  - 3 The caruncle
- B Fat pad

The plica semilunaris is located far medially in the palpebral fissure and is predominantly below the midline. The caruncle is located medial to the plica. It is covered with squamous epithelium and often contains small hairs. The relationships of the plica and caruncle to each other and to the palpebral fissure are important cosmetic factors in strabismus surgery. When incising and repairing conjunctiva, care should be taken to leave the position of the plica and caruncle undisturbed. It is particularly important that the plica not be displaced laterally, making it more obvious as a reddened unsightly mass in the palpebral fissure.

Anterior to the inferior fornix, a fat pad is present that extends to within 12 to 14 mm of the limbus. This fat pad is beneath the conjunctiva and its posterior condensations and is outside both layers of Tenon's capsule. A transconjunctival incision made medially or laterally should be made posterior to the line of attachment of posterior Tenon's capsule or at least 8 mm from the limbus but anterior to the inferior fat pad or no more than 12 mm from the limbus.

During extraocular muscle surgery, incisions should be limited to bulbar conjunctiva and should not extend into the fornix or palpebral conjunctiva.* This causes unnecessary bleeding and serves no purpose.

In cases where prior surgery has left the conjunctiva reddened and unsightly or scarred so that it limits motility, the conjunctiva may be recessed with or without removal of tissue. When this is done, sclera should be left uncovered. The sclera quickly becomes recovered with epithelium, and the use of a mucous membrane graft is unnecessary.

---

*The Parks cul-de-sac or fornix incision for exposure of the extraocular muscles is actually made in bulbar conjunctiva.

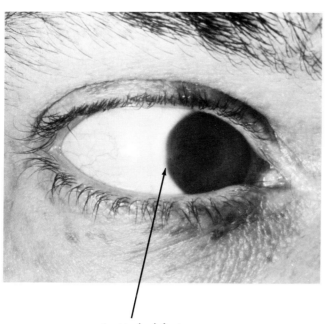

A

1. Limbal fusion

2. Plica semilunaris

3. Caruncle

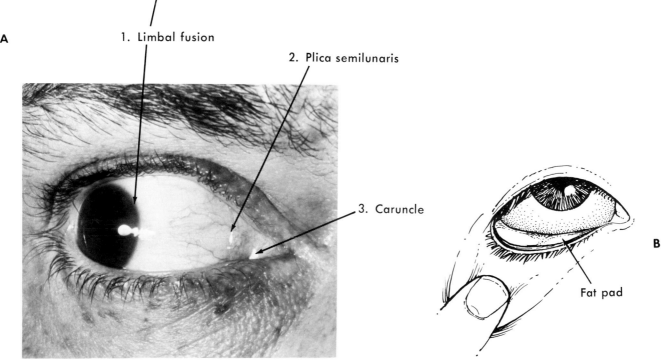

B

Fat pad

PLATE 1-4

9

TENON'S CAPSULE

Tenon's capsule is a thick structure with definite body and substance in childhood, but it gradually atrophies until in old age it is fibrillar and fragile. It is divided into anterior and posterior parts. Anterior Tenon's capsule is the vestigial capsulopalpebral head of the rectus muscles.* This structure overlies the anterior half to two thirds of the rectus muscles as well as the intermuscular space and membrane and fuses with the conjunctiva at the limbus. Anterior to the line of insertion of the rectus muscles, a potential space exists between conjunctiva and anterior Tenon's capsule and also between anterior Tenon's capsule and sclera.

Posterior Tenon's capsule is composed of the fibrous sheath of the rectus muscles together with the intermuscular membrane. According to Lester T. Jones, the sheaths that make up posterior Tenon's capsule form at a later evolutionary stage than those forming anterior Tenon's capsule. Fibrous attachments between the inner surface of anterior Tenon's capsule and the outer muscle sheath (part of posterior Tenon's capsule) are called "check ligaments." Other attachments between the outer surface of anterior Tenon's capsule and the orbital rim medially and laterally are also called check ligaments. Most extraocular muscle surgery is done beneath anterior Tenon's capsule in the plane of posterior Tenon's capsule (because the intermuscular membrane must be severed to some extent). Retinal detachment surgery is done beneath posterior Tenon's capsule. A free space exists beneath posterior Tenon's capsule except for the point of exit of the vortex veins and the point of entrance of the posterior ciliary arteries and nerves.

PLATE 1-5

A 1 Medial wall of the orbit
  2 Fibrous attachments between anterior Tenon's capsule, the wall of the orbit, and orbital fat
  3 Anterior Tenon's capsule
  4 Fibrous attachments between anterior Tenon's capsule and the muscle sheath (posterior Tenon's capsule)
  5 The muscle in its sheath (posterior Tenon's capsule)
  6 Intermuscular membrane (posterior Tenon's capsule)
  7 Orbital fat

B 1 The limbal fusion of conjunctiva and anterior Tenon's capsule
  2 Potential space between anterior Tenon's capsule and sclera
  3 The muscle in its sheath (posterior Tenon's capsule) inserting into sclera
  4 Postinsertional muscle footplates
  5 Episclera

C Coronal section of B at X

1	Conjunctiva	4	Extraocular muscle
2	Anterior Tenon's capsule	5	Intermuscular membrane
3	Muscle sheath	6	Sclera

*Lester T. Jones suggests that anterior and posterior Tenon's capsule are separate structures formed at different evolutionary stages. (Trans. Am. Acad. Ophthalmol. Otolaryngol. 72[5]:755-764, 1968.)

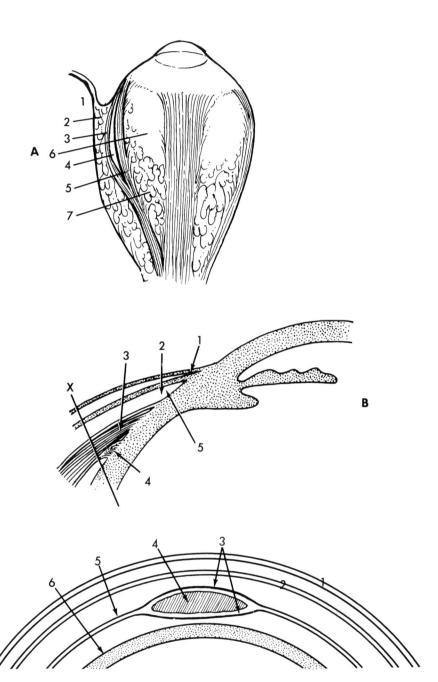

PLATE 1-5

Ant tenon's Capsule inserts at limbus
Post tenon's Capsule inserts at the line of insertion of recti.

TENON'S CAPSULE—cont'd

The separateness of anterior and posterior Tenon's capsule can be appreciated when approach to the rectus muscle is made with a limbal incision. The limbal incision first incises fused conjunctiva—anterior Tenon's capsule at the limbus, allowing these layers to be retracted as a unit and exposing the muscle encased in its sheath.

PLATE 1-6

A When the layer of combined conjunctiva–anterior Tenon's capsule is retracted, the muscle insertion in its sheath is exposed. Fibrous attachments are seen and the fusion of the intermuscular membrane (posterior Tenon's capsule) to sclera is apparent. This fusion of intermuscular membrane to sclera must be incised before bare sclera and posterior Tenon's space can be encountered. Only after entering subposterior Tenon's space can the insertion of the rectus muscle be engaged cleanly on a muscle hook. This is the "free space" used by the retina surgeon.

B The insertion of posterior Tenon's capsule rings the globe at the level of the rectus muscle insertions. Between this insertion and the limbus, sclera is covered by episclera, which may be a forward extension of posterior Tenon's capsule, anterior Tenon's capsule, and conjunctiva.

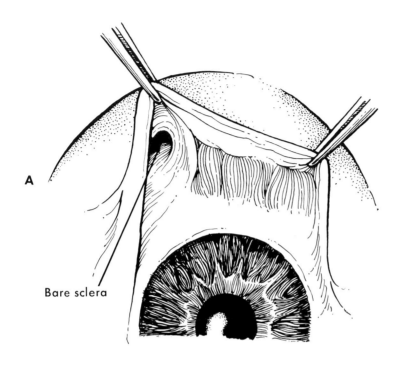

A

Bare sclera

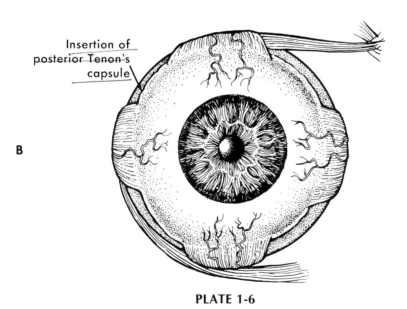

Insertion of
posterior Tenon's
capsule

B

PLATE 1-6

THE RECTUS MUSCLES

Each rectus muscle inserts at a different distance from the limbus. This point of insertion is the most important landmark of extraocular muscle surgery.

The medial rectus inserts 5.5 mm from the limbus (range: 3 to 6 mm). I have measured the distance between the medial rectus muscle insertion and the limbus of 112 medial rectus muscles in 66 esotropic patients. The average distance of the medial rectus muscle from the limbus was 4.4 mm. Eight patients had unequal insertion distances. There was no correlation between the angle of the deviation and the distance of the medial rectus muscle from the limbus. The variability of this insertion makes it a poor landmark for measuring when doing a recession. For this reason I now use the limbus as the point of reference for recession of the medial rectus muscles. Of course, the amount of recession must be adjusted when measuring from the limbus. The inferior rectus inserts 6.5 mm from the limbus, the lateral rectus inserts 6.9 mm from the limbus (range: 4.5 to 8 mm), and the superior rectus inserts 7.7 mm from the limbus. Beginning with the medial rectus and going inferiorly and temporally, each rectus muscle inserts farther from the limbus. This is called the spiral of Tillaux.

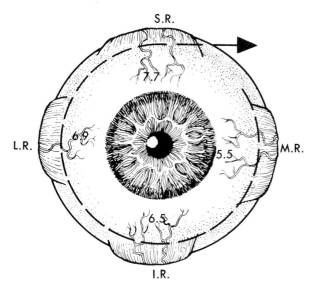

PLATE 1-7

THE RECTUS MUSCLES—cont'd

The insertion of the rectus muscles in most instances can be seen through the intact conjunctiva.

When the eye is rotated and the conjunctiva is brought tightly over the insertion of any of the rectus muscles, close observation will reveal the line of insertion of the muscle, as indicated by the dotted line in the figure. Such observation allows the surgeon to locate accurately the 3, 6, 9, and 12 o'clock positions of the globe. This maneuver for orientation leads to proper traction suture placement and ensures accurate placement of the conjunctival incision and accurate localization of the muscle to be operated upon.

The rectus muscles are all approximately 40 mm in length and receive their innervation at the junction of the posterior and middle thirds of the muscles, or approximately 26 mm from their insertion. Dimensions and points of innervation of all the extraocular muscles are listed in Table 1.

Table 1. Extraocular muscles

Muscle	Length (mm)	Nerve	Point of innervation	Tendon* (mm)
Medial rectus (MR)	40	III Inferior division	26 mm from insertion	L: 3.7 W: 10.3
Inferior rectus (IR)	40	III Inferior division	26 mm from insertion	L: 5.5 W: 9.8
Lateral rectus (LR)	40	VI	26 mm from insertion	L: 8.8 W: 9.2
Superior rectus (SR)	40	III Superior division	26 mm from insertion	L: 5.8 W: 10.8
Inferior oblique (IO)	36	III Inferior division	12 mm posterior to insertion of inferior rectus at its lateral border	L: < 1 W: 9.4
Superior oblique (SO)	60	IV	26 mm from trochlea	L: 30 W: 10.7

*L, Length; W, width.

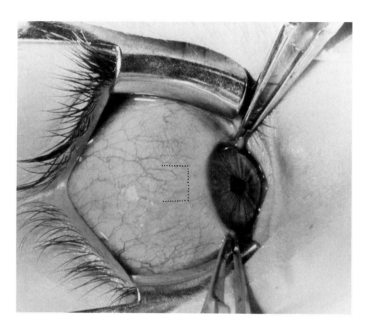

PLATE 1-8

THE INFERIOR OBLIQUE

PLATE 1-9

A The inferior oblique muscle is 36 mm long. It originates near the medial end of the inferior orbital rim at the outer crest of the lacrimal fossa and proceeds posteriorly and temporally at an angle of 50 degrees, with the frontal plane going beneath the inferior rectus (between the inferior rectus and the floor of the orbit). It inserts beneath the inferior border of the lateral rectus muscle, approximately 12 mm from the insertion of the lateral rectus. The posterior extent of the inferior oblique insertion is 2 mm below and 2 mm lateral to the macula, and the proximal one third of the distal half of the muscle overlies the inferior temporal vortex vein. The blood vessels in the inferior oblique do not contribute to the blood supply of the anterior segment of the globe. This muscle receives its innervation on its upper surface at the point where it passes beneath the lateral border of the inferior rectus, approximately 12 mm posterior to the insertion of the inferior rectus. The inferior oblique muscle is unique in its anatomic relationships. This muscle behaves as though it has two potential insertions and two potential points of origin. Since the inferior oblique is innervated near its middle, it may be weakened either proximal or distal to its point of innervation.

B A weakening procedure of the inferior oblique done lateral to the lateral border of the inferior rectus causes the new functional insertion of the inferior oblique to be at its point of union with Lockwood's ligament beneath the inferior rectus. The origin remains at the crest of the lacrimal fossa.

C A weakening procedure of the inferior oblique done medial to the medial border of the inferior rectus* causes the new point of origin for the inferior oblique to be at its point of union with Lockwood's ligament. The insertion remains at a point below and temporal to the macula.

Because of these unique anatomic relationships, a disinsertion, myectomy, or large recession of the inferior oblique muscle may be done without crippling it.

---

*This technique for weakening the inferior oblique is unpredictable and should not be done. The anatomic relationship has theoretical interest only.

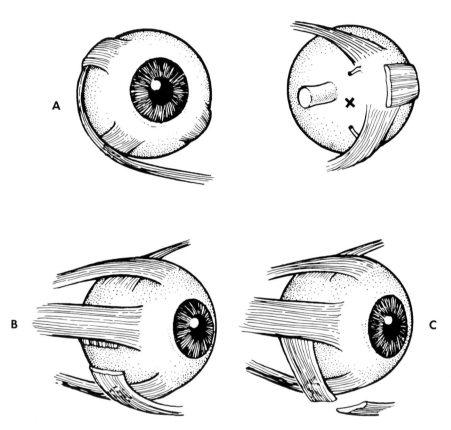

PLATE 1-9

THE SUPERIOR OBLIQUE

PLATE 1-10

A   The superior oblique muscle has a muscular portion and a tendinous portion, both of which are 30 mm long. The muscle, which originates at the annulus of Zinn, becomes tendinous 10 mm before reaching the trochlea, a cartilaginous tunnel located at the junction of the medial and superior orbital rim just posterior to the orbital rim. The trochlea acts as a pulley. The tendinous portion of the superior oblique goes through the trochlea and then courses posteriorly and temporally at approximately 54° from the frontal plane. It passes beneath the superior rectus to insert near the lateral border of the superior rectus. The average anterior point of insertion of the superior oblique tendon is approximately 13 mm from the limbus. The superior oblique tendon between the trochlea and the medial border of the superior rectus is about 3 mm in diameter, white, and is surrounded by dense fascia. Because of this fascia, the superior oblique tendon medial to the superior rectus can be somewhat difficult to identify. However, when the fascia is dissected, the superior oblique tendon is an easily distinguishable structure. The nerve to the superior oblique enters the muscular portion 26 mm posterior to the trochlea. There are no blood vessels in the superior oblique that contribute to the blood supply of the anterior segment of the globe.

B   The insertion of the superior oblique is broad, measuring an average of 10.7 mm. The superior oblique is the most variable of the extraocular muscles in that it may insert at varying distances from the limbus. It is often found inserting greater than 13.0 mm from the limbus, but it is usually near the lateral border of the superior rectus. However, I attempted a superior oblique tuck on a patient with congenital underaction of the superior oblique and was unable to find the tendinous insertion at either the lateral border of or beneath the superior rectus. The superior oblique tendon was then isolated medial to the superior rectus and was traced posteriorly, remaining *medial* to the superior rectus. To avoid the possibility of interference with the posterior ciliary vessels and nerves, the actual insertion was not identified. In this case the middle portion of the superior oblique tendon was sutured to sclera at the lateral border of the superior rectus 12 mm from the limbus without tucking or severing the tendon. On three occasions I have attempted superior oblique tucks on patients, who after careful, thorough dissections were found to have no superior oblique tendon.

C   Whitnall's (superior transverse) ligament and the superior oblique tendon have common fascial attachments near the trochlea. If the superior transverse ligament is weakened inadvertently while hooking the superior oblique tendon, thereby weakening the medial horn of the levator muscle, ptosis of the nasal portion of the upper lid may result. For this reason, it is safer to hook the superior oblique tendon under direct vision and preferably at its insertion.

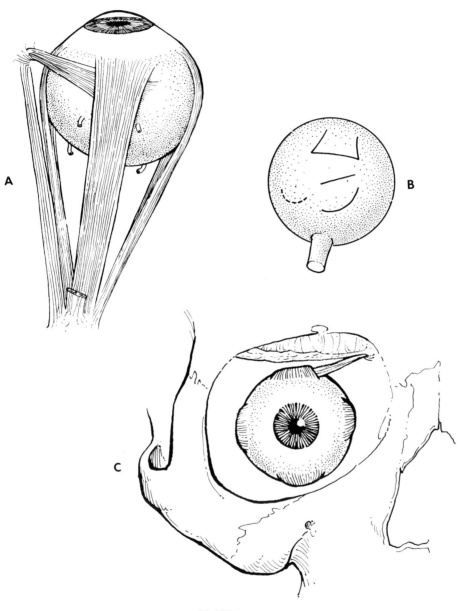

PLATE 1-10

21

THE BLOOD SUPPLY

PLATE 1-11

A The principal blood supply to the anterior segment of the eye comes through the anterior ciliary arteries, which travel in the four rectus muscles. Each of the rectus muscles has two anterior ciliary arteries, with the exception of the lateral rectus, which has one. As a general rule, not more than two rectus muscles should be detached at one operation, and if two adjacent rectus muscles are detached at one operation in an older individual, segmental iris atrophy may occur. If two rectus muscles are detached (horizontal recession-resection), a period of 2 months or more should elapse before surgery is done on the other rectus muscles. There are exceptions to this rule (see Chapter 11).

B The four vortex veins are located behind the equator a few millimeters on each side of the superior and inferior rectus muscles. A vortex vein may be encountered during any type of extraocular muscle surgery, but the most common times are during inferior or superior rectus recession and resection, inferior oblique weakening, and exposure of the superior oblique insertion. Every effort should be made to avoid severing a vortex vein. If a vortex vein is cut, pressure should be applied to control bleeding. Cautery should be avoided.

22

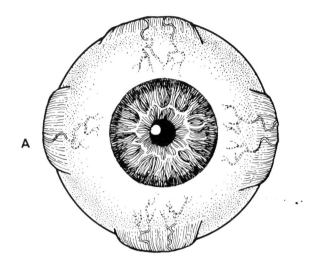

A

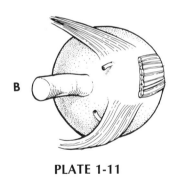

B

PLATE 1-11

23

THE SCLERA

PLATE 1-12

A The thickness of the sclera varies.
1 At the limbus the sclera is 0.8 mm thick.
2 Anterior to the rectus muscle insertions it is 0.6 mm thick.
3 Posterior to the rectus muscle insertions it is 0.3 mm thick.
4 At the equator it is 0.5 mm thick.
5 At the posterior pole it is greater than 1 mm thick.

The area of greatest surgical activity for the extraocular muscle surgeon coincides with the thinnest area of the sclera.

B Care must be exercised when placing a needle into sclera.
1 A reverse cutting needle should be used with extreme caution because such a needle may be as thick or thicker than the sclera into which it is inserted. This could lead to scleral perforation, an event that undoubtedly occurs more often than is suspected or reported. If such a cutting needle is used, it should be very fine (less than 0.3 mm), and it should be inserted carefully with the top of the needle seen through superficial sclera at all times.
2 A curved cutting needle is less likely to perforate sclera than a reverse cutting needle, but the curved cutting needle is prone to cut itself out of sclera unless an excessively deep bite is taken.
3 A much safer needle to use is the spatula design. With such a needle, only the tip and sides are cutting edges. Sclera is *displaced* upward and downward and *cut* laterally and ahead of the needle. This makes the complication of scleral perforation less likely to occur with spatula needles than with reverse cutting needles provided the spatula needle's widest dimension remains parallel to the scleral surface.

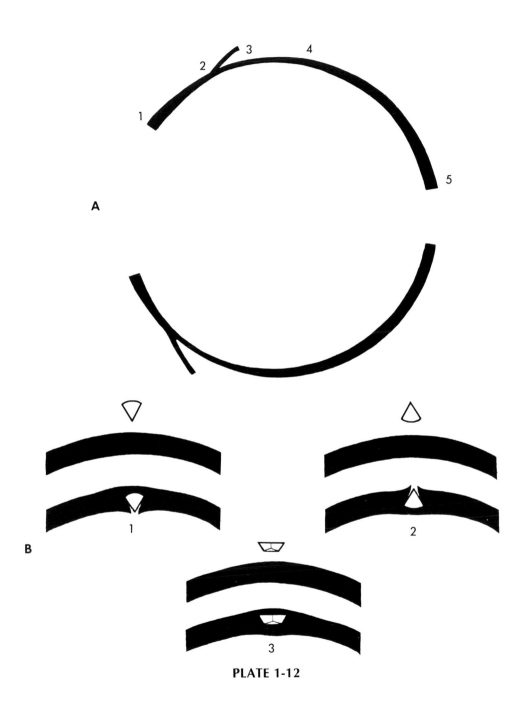

A

B

1

2

3

PLATE 1-12

CHAPTER TWO

Instrumentation, anesthesia, preparation of the patient for surgery, and postoperative care

The instruments required for extraocular muscle surgery are simple in nature and few in number. But, as with any type of surgery, it is essential that the surgeon have available to him all of the instruments he might require for a particular procedure and that these instruments be in good working order.

Anesthesia suitable for extraocular muscle surgery varies with the patient's individual requirements and also with the surgeon's personal preference. Children always require general anesthesia with either endotracheal intubation, insufflation, or dissociation. The general anesthetic agent or agents used are usually determined by the anesthesiologist. Cooperative adults may be operated upon successfully with local anesthesia, and a few surgeons prefer topical anesthesia for extraocular muscle surgery in carefully selected patients.

Preparation of the patient for surgery in the operating room prior to extraocular muscle surgery requires only that the lids and face around both eyes be washed and properly draped and that the operative field be free of clutter.

Patches and/or antibiotic drops or ointment with or without steroids may be utilized according to the surgeon's preference.

INSTRUMENTS USED IN STRABISMUS SURGERY

The complete instrument assortment for strabismus surgery is shown as it is assembled on the surgery stand. Of course, not every instrument is used in each case, but we routinely include the complete set of the instruments for every case. The instruments are arranged approximately in the same order used during the procedure. The instruments should be assembled in the same way for every case and should be kept clean and maintained in an orderly fashion throughout the procedure.

PLATE 2-1

Bottom row from left to right:
    Silk traction suture, 4-0 or 5-0
    Plain collagen suture, 5-0 (or the surgeon's choice for conjunctival closure)
    5-0 or 6-0 braided Vicryl with an "S"-14 or "S"-24 needle (or the surgeon's choice for muscle reattachment)
    Bard-Parker handle with No. 15 blade
    Spring action blunt tip scissors (Wescott)
    Utility forceps (Thorpe) (3)
    Utility forceps (Nugent)
    Strabismus (muscle) hook (6)
        Culler hook (1)
        Jameson hook (1)
        von Graefe hook (1)
        Steven's hook (3)
    Smooth tying forceps (2)
    Tendon tucker (Bishop)

Middle row from left to right:
    Self-adhering aperture drape
    Lid speculums
        Infant
        Child
        Adult
    Serrefine (2)
    Electrocautery (Scheie) (battery not shown) or disposable cautery

Top row from left to right:
    Sterile eye pad (2)
    Angled marginal myotomy hemostats (Helveston's design)
    Caliper
    Retractor (Desmarres) (small)
    Resection clamps (Jameson) (4)
        Adult (right and left)
        Child (right and left)
    Needle holder (Castroviejo), heavy model (2)
    Mosquito hemostats (2)

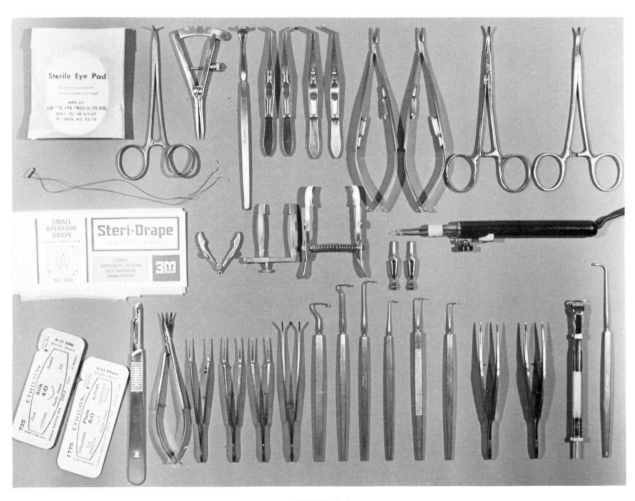

PLATE 2-1

ANESTHESIA FOR STRABISMUS SURGERY

The type of anesthesia (general, dissociative, local, or topical) chosen for strabismus surgery is dictated by the requirements of the patient and modified by the preference and experience of the surgeon. If general anesthesia is the choice, the anesthesiologist then decides upon the specific agent or agents to be used as well as the amount and type of premedication. However, in patients in whom echothiophate iodide (Phospholine Iodide) has been employed, the use of succinylcholine is definitely contraindicated. A patient who has been treated with echothiophate iodide can retain low blood levels of cholinesterase for weeks or even months after discontinuing the medicine. In the presence of low blood cholinesterase, succinylcholine causes prolonged apnea that may require the patient to be assisted by a respirator for several hours after surgery to ensure proper ventilation. Because of this danger, I avoid the use of succinylcholine in children undergoing strabismus surgery.

General anesthesia

Most immature patients (younger than the midteens) require general anesthesia for extraocular muscle surgery. This anesthetic may be administered through an endotracheal tube, with the anesthetic agent and oxygen being delivered directly to the lungs, or by insufflation, a system where the patient breathes the anesthetic agent or agents along with room air. The agent most commonly used for general anesthesia is halothane (Fluothane). Other agents such as fluroxene (Fluoromar), cyclopropane, methoxyflurane (Penthrane), and a combination of nitrous oxide, barbiturate, and narcotics may be used but have no advantage over halothane. Thiopental sodium (Pentothal Sodium) given intravenously or nitrous oxide given by mask are the most common agents used for induction prior to intubation. Open drop ether may also be used for induction and maintenance of anesthesia in infants. Ether has a wide margin of safety but postoperative vomiting is frequent. Preoperative medication for infants should be limited to a moderate dose of atropine given intramuscularly. Older children and adults having general anesthesia require narcotics and, in some cases, barbiturates in addition to atropine. The doses should, of course, be individualized.

With more outpatient strabismus surgery now being done, it is important to avoid the use of, or at least reduce the amount of, narcotics and barbiturates given to children preoperatively. The advantage of being able to use a slightly reduced amount of general anesthetic agent after premedication with narcotics is more than outweighed by the fact that after a short procedure a heavily premedicated patient may exhibit prolonged drowsiness not from the general anesthetic agent but from the preoperative medications.

General anesthesia allows the surgeon more complete freedom in manipulation of the muscles and allows accurate interpretation of forced ductions. Many surgeons prefer general anesthesia for all strabismus surgery for these reasons. As with general anesthesia used for any type of surgery, patients undergoing strabismus surgery should be monitored constantly by the anesthesiologist to diagnose emergencies such as arrhythmias, the bradycardia associated with the oculocardiac reflex, or cardiac arrest immediately. When bradycardia occurs, all manipulation of the muscle should stop immediately and the muscle should not be touched again until the heart rate returns to normal. If repeated muscle stimulation causes further bradycardia, the patient should be given intravenous atropine by the anesthesiologist. Bradycardia persisting after atropine has been injected intravenously may be treated with a retrobulbar injection of 3 to 5 ml of 1% or 2% lidocaine (Xylocaine). Cardiac arrest is treated with ventilation, and closed chest heart massage is begun *immediately*. If cardiac contraction does not begin after several minutes, 3 to 5 ml of intravenous epinephrine 1:10,000 may be given.

In the Indiana University Clinic, patients undergoing strabismus surgery who are otherwise healthy and have intelligent, cooperative parents may be admitted to the hospital the morning of surgery and discharged the same afternoon. Parents are told ahead of time that if any complications should arise postoperatively, the patient will be kept in the hospital overnight following surgery. The length of hospital stay for patients who have strabismus surgery is determined almost entirely by their ability to recover from anesthesia.

Dissociative anesthesia

Ketamine, a new dissociative anesthetic agent, has been used recently for a variety of ophthalmic procedures including strabismus surgery. With ketamine the patient has no cognizance of pain because the drug causes a dissociation between the painful stimulus and any awareness of this stimulus. Purposeless movements of all parts of the body, including the eyes, do persist with ketamine, and tonus of the extraocular muscles remains. For these reasons the eye must be anchored with traction sutures and the surgeon must be constantly alert for unexpected ocular movements. The persistent tonus also makes interpretation of forced ductions less reliable.

In older children and adults, prolonged drowsiness accompanied by disturbing dreams and hallucinations are a significant drawback to the use of ketamine. I used ketamine for forty-four consecutive surgical procedures, thirty-three of which were strabismus procedures, and concluded that ketamine was generally unsatisfactory for strabismus surgery.

Local anesthesia

Either 1% or 2% lidocaine (Xylocaine) with or without epinephrine 1:100,000 added provides satisfactory anesthesia for strabismus surgery in cooperative teenagers and adults. From 2 to 3 ml of the agent is injected subcutaneously into the upper and lower lids just inside the orbital rim to anesthetize and paralyze the lids. From 3 to 5 ml of the same agent is then injected into the retrobulbar space (into the muscle cone) and after a wait of 5 minutes surgery may begin. A well-done retrobulbar injection with lidocaine gives satisfactory anesthesia to the anterior globe and extraocular muscles. However, the patient may experience pain deep in the orbit, presumably in the area of annulus of Zinn, when muscles are tugged upon, particularly during a resection procedure. Patients also may experience pain when the insertion of a muscle is manipulated. In general, a surgeon must exercise more care in performing surgery under local anesthesia. If the surgeon prefers to avoid doing a retrobulbar injection, local infiltration with lidocaine around the muscle's insertion as well as subconjunctivally in the quadrants above and below the muscle can be effective. Care must be taken,

31

however, to exert very little traction on the extraocular muscles because of the pain that this maneuver produces.

Topical anesthesia

After a lid block has been obtained as described previously, surgery may be performed on the extraocular muscles of a cooperative adult using only 5% proparacaine hydrochloride (Ophthaine) and 5% cocaine hydrochloride solution instilled in the cul-de-sacs and repeatedly on the operative site. Such a technique demands an extremely cooperative patient and therefore has limited application. Those who advocate use of topical anesthesia claim that prism and cover testing may be done at the time of surgery with the patient either lying on the table or sitting up. Results obtained from surgery are said to be better because of this "on the table" testing, which allows adjustments in the amount of surgery done in such cases. Because few patients are stoic enough to withstand the rigors of topical anesthesia, it is doubtful that this technique will ever reach widespread use.

PREPARATION OF THE PATIENT IN THE OPERATING ROOM

PLATE 2-2

A The patient should be positioned so that his head is at the very end of the operating table. The surrounding area should be free of unnecessary equipment. If general anesthesia is used, connectors should be fashioned so that tubes will not interfere with the field. Even though the endotracheal tube is well anchored, the surgeon should always warn the anesthesiologist before moving the head. When insufflation anesthesia is used the anesthesiologist must be able to observe the patient's breathing. Use of insufflation anesthesia requires an expert anesthesiologist and a high degree of cooperation between the anesthesiologist and the surgeon.

B A disposable head immobilizer is a convenient device for stabilizing the head during surgery. An adult size fits adults and older children. An infant size is also available.

C After anesthesia has been obtained, the area around both eyes should be washed thoroughly. My technique is to wash the skin in the area outlined using pHisoHex and water for 3 to 5 minutes. This is followed by a thorough rinse with sterile water. Care should be taken to prevent soap from getting into the cul-de-sacs and onto the corneas. To avoid painful pHisoHex keratitis, any soap that does get onto the cornea or into the cul-de-sacs should be removed promptly and thoroughly with a sterile saline rinse. Two drops of Argyrol are then placed in each cul-de-sac to precipitate the mucoid secretions. The cul-de-sacs are then rinsed with sterile normal saline. Ioprep is painted over the area that has been scrubbed and the skin is blotted dry. Before draping is completed, forced ductions are done in *all* directions in *both* eyes. The eyelashes are not trimmed.

D Cloth drapes are placed over the nose, forehead, and sides of the head, and the self-adhering operative drape is positioned. The unencumbered field illustrated is ideal for extraocular muscle surgery.

32

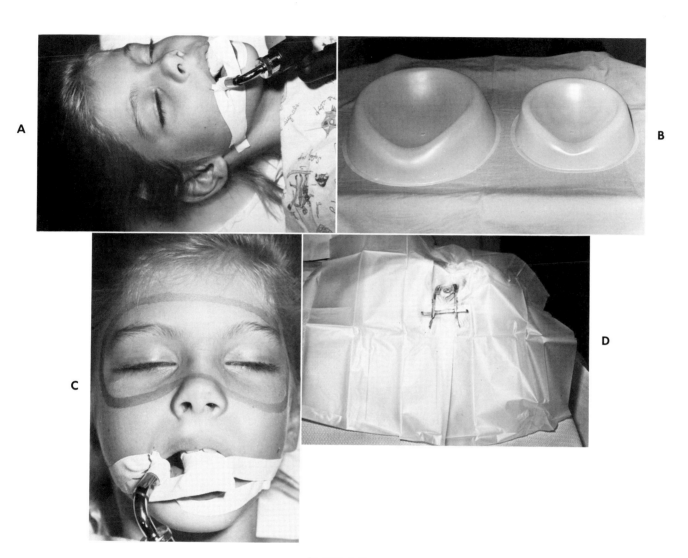

PLATE 2-2

POSTOPERATIVE CARE OF THE PATIENT

A patch may be used postoperatively, but never over both eyes. Any questionable benefit resulting from reduced ocular motility is far outweighed by the emotional trauma caused by bilateral patching. If both eyes have been operated upon with a single muscle done on each eye, no patch is used. If a recession-resection has been done on one eye, a patch may be placed over the operated eye for 24 hours and then is discontinued. If three or more muscles are done with both eyes operated upon, the eye with greater reaction may be patched for 24 hours only. I use a patch in fewer than 5% of all strabismus patients who undergo surgery.

As with patching, the use of drops or ointments postoperatively varies from surgeon to surgeon. Some prefer none while others use antibiotic drops or ointment and still others use antibiotics and steroids in combination. My routine is to use an ointment with sodium sulfacetamide and prednisolone combined twice a day for 3 days, then once a day for 1 week.

Patients are seen during the afternoon following surgery and ocular motility is checked. These so-called trouble rounds are made primarily to observe the variety of early postoperative alignments that may occur in similar patients who have received similar surgery and to ensure proper muscle attachment by noting movement of the operated eye (see Chapter 12). Patients are discharged the day of surgery or the following morning. Three days postoperatively the patients are checked as outpatients. They are seen again 10 days and 6 weeks postoperatively. At the 6 weeks' visit the results of surgery are usually apparent. In cases where early postoperative treatment such as prisms, patching, echothiophate iodide, or other techniques are necessary, the postoperative routine is individualized according to the patients' needs.

CHAPTER THREE

Sutures, sleeves, implantation material, and adhesives

SUTURES FOR EXTRAOCULAR MUSCLE SURGERY
Absorbable sutures

The most popular type of suture for most extraocular muscle surgery has been absorbable—either catgut or collagen, plain or chromic—and varies in size from 4-0 to 6-0. Catgut differs from collagen in that the former is made from individual sheep intestines, which are composed of 95% collagen and 5% noncollagenous associated tissue. On the other hand, collagen sutures are formed by an extrusion of homogenized, pooled, beef fascia and are 100% collagen. Theoretically the pooled tissue making up collagen sutures should cause it to have reduced antigenicity, but my experience has been that the incidence of mild acute allergic reaction and chronic suture granuloma formation is the same when using catgut or collagen sutures (19% mild acute suture reaction and 0.5% chronic suture granuloma). Collagen sutures have better tying qualities than catgut sutures because collagen is more conformable. Collagen ties into a more secure knot with less memory effect (tendency to straighten) than catgut, so untying is less likely to occur.

The size of the suture used for recession and resection is dictated by the surgeon's preference rather than by an established set of rules. The same is also true regarding the use of chromic versus plain suture. In general, however, the handling and holding properties of chromic suture tend to make it a bit stronger than plain suture of the same size. As a minimum, 6-0 chromic catgut or collagen may be used for recession or resection. Seldom, if ever, is suture heavier than 4-0 chromic collagen or catgut required for strabismus surgery.

New synthetic absorbable sutures made of glycolic acid polymers have the advantage of being strong and essentially nonantigenic. Their disadvantages are that they produce tissue drag because of their braided design and that they become stiff when exposed. My preference for muscle reattachment when absorbable suture is required is 5-0 or 6-0 braided Polyglactin 910 sutures with a spatula needle. For conjunctival closure I prefer 5-0 plain collagen with a spatula needle. In my opinion synthetic absorbable sutures are far superior to animal-product sutures for buried use.

35

TECHNIQUES FOR HANDLING SYNTHETIC ABSORBABLE SUTURE

PLATE 3-1

Tissue adherence and premature knotting are complications that may occur when using synthetic absorbable suture. These can be eliminated or reduced by the use of proper technique.

A Synthetic absorbable suture that is braided has a tendency to "grab" fascia as the suture is drawn across the globe. This extraneous tissue should be pulled free before tying the knot that secures the muscle to the globe. Running the suture through moistened gloved fingers before using helps to smooth the suture's surface and reduces its tendency to grab.

B Synthetic absorbable suture can knot prematurely if excess pressure is applied while bringing the knot down. To avoid this premature knotting, the surgeon should avoid applying tension to the knot as it slides down to the point where it is to be secured. Only when the knot is brought down to the tissue should the suture be pulled taut.

Nonabsorbable sutures

A variety of nonabsorbable sutures have been found useful for extraocular muscle surgery. These include silk, nylon, Merseline, Dacron, Supramid Extra, and even stainless steel. Some surgeons prefer to use 5-0 or 6-0 nonabsorbable sutures for recession and resection procedures. However, nonabsorbable suture materials are subject to early and late extrusion and can serve as the nidus for granuloma or abscess formation. Proper technique when using nonabsorbable sutures is essential. When such sutures are used in recession or resection, the knots are much less likely to extrude if they are tied beneath the muscle as described by Reinecke (see p. 70).

Nonabsorbable sutures such as 5-0 or 6-0 Merseline, nylon, silk, or Dacron should be used in muscle or tendon tucking procedures of the superior oblique, inferior oblique, or rectus muscles. They should also be used for joining the muscle bellies in the muscle transposition procedure described by Jensen. In each instance the sutures are placed well posterior and extrusion is seldom a problem. In such cases, even when late extrusion does occur, the results of surgery seem stable. Nonabsorbable sutures should also be used for anchoring Supramid sheets.

The 4-0 or 5-0 black silk sutures placed into the episclera near the limbus are useful but not essential for immobilizing and retracting the eye during surgery. These 4-0 or 5-0 black silk sutures are also useful as traction sutures to fix the globe in a given position for several days postoperatively in cases where surgery is done to correct mechanical restriction.

Several 8-0 white silk sutures may be used for closure of the limbal incision. These sutures usually extrude harmlessly but occasionally must be removed.

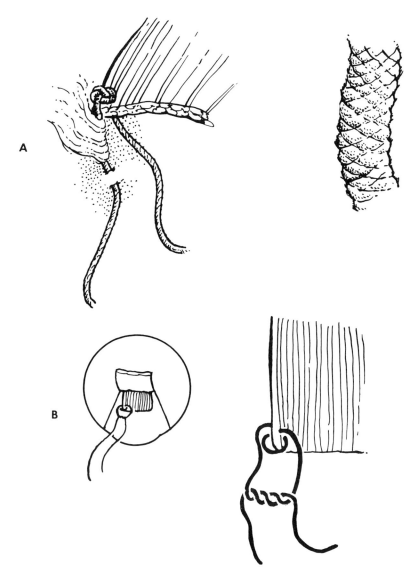

A

B

PLATE 3-1

NEEDLES

The safest needles for extraocular muscle surgery are of the fine spatula design. The spatula needle cuts tissue at its tip and sides only and actually displaces tissue above and below. This results in less chance of inadvertent scleral perforation, provided the flat of the spatula is parallel to the sclera. Curved cutting and reverse cutting needles, if employed, should be used with caution and should be of very fine caliber. At the present time only reverse cutting needles are available on 4-0 black silk, which is frequently used for placement of traction sutures, so extra care should be employed when using this material.

PLASTIC SLEEVES, IMPLANTS, AND ADHESIVES
Sleeves

To reduce the detrimental effect on motility caused by scarring and adhesion formation, particularly in repeat extraocular muscle surgery and extraocular muscle surgery for restriction, Dunlap has devised sleeves made of Supramid Extra that fit over the muscle. These sleeves form a smooth, inert tunnel within which the muscle may contract and relax uninfluenced by scarring of adjacent tissue. These sleeves are 0.05 mm thick and 15.0 mm long and are available in diameters of 4.0, 5.0, and 7.0 mm.

Implants

Supramid Extra sheets, which are 0.05 mm thick, are available in 4 × 6 inch sheets and in partial spheres that encompass one eighth to one quarter of the globe. These are placed between the sclera and muscle and between the muscle and anterior Tenon's capsule in cases where whole quadrants of the globe are involved in scar formation. Gelfilm has been used widely in the past but is not effective in preventing adhesion formation and should *not* be used.

Adhesives

Cyanoacrylate adhesives were first studied to determine their usefulness in gluing extraocular muscles to sclera. The results were disappointing and at present adhesives are not clinically useful in strabismus surgery. An interesting alternative use of adhesives is that when properly applied they can form a protective coat around muscles or upon sclera. This coat serves as a barrier against adhesion formation. At the present time the use of adhesives in extraocular muscle surgery remains experimental.

Various materials such as silicone and Supramid Extra have been tried for tendon lengthening. These procedures remain experimental.

CHAPTER FOUR

Techniques of exposure

THE CONJUNCTIVAL INCISION

Three basic techniques have been described for the incision through conjunctiva to gain surgical exposure to the extraocular muscles. They differ primarily in their location relative to the palpebral opening. All three, however, stress the importance of operating on the muscles *beneath* anterior Tenon's capsule to disturb anterior Tenon's capsule as little as possible, thereby reducing the likelihood of postoperative adhesion formation between anterior Tenon's capsule and the muscle sheath. The value of extraocular muscle surgery performed *beneath* anterior Tenon's capsule was first pointed out by Swan.

The three techniques are:

1. The transconjunctival incision in the palpebral opening (Swan)
2. The transconjunctival incision in the cul-de-sac (Parks)
3. The limbal incision in the palpebral opening (popularized in the United States by von Noorden)

A slight modification of the transconjunctival incision in the cul-de-sac (retropalpebral-transconjunctival) is useful in gaining exposure to the oblique muscles.

The initial surgical exposure of the extraocular muscles while still in their sheaths is accomplished after an incision has been made through conjunctiva and anterior Tenon's capsule only. In order for the insertion of the rectus muscle to be engaged on a muscle hook *cleanly,* the intermuscular membrane must then be incised and bare sclera exposed. Before any attempt is made to "hook" an extraocular muscle, the tip of the muscle hook must be placed on *bare sclera,* slipped cleanly behind the insertion of the muscle, and then identified at the muscle's opposite border.

THE CONJUNCTIVAL INCISION—cont'd

Either the transconjunctival, cul-de-sac, or limbal approach may be used for exposure of any of the *rectus muscles*. The incision of choice for exposing the *oblique muscles* when they are operated upon alone is transconjunctival and behind the lids.

The perfect incision for operation on the extraocular muscles would fulfill the following requirements:

1. Minimal scar visible in the palpebral fissure after surgery
2. Adequate exposure
3. Ease of performance
4. Lack of postoperative adhesion formation between Tenon's capsule, muscle sheath, and sclera
5. Ease of reoperation
6. Relaxation of tight, restrictive conjunctiva and anterior Tenon's capsule.

No single incision for exposing the extraocular muscles fulfills all of these requirements, but my choice for most procedures done on the horizontal rectus muscles is the limbal incision.

PLATE 4-1

A   The transconjunctival incision of Swan is made slightly behind the insertion of the medial or lateral rectus muscle (6.5 mm from the limbus for medial rectus exposure and 7.9 mm from the limbus for lateral rectus exposure) and is as wide as the muscle itself (approximately 10 mm).

B   The cul-de-sac incision is made approximately 4 mm above or below the limbus and extends approximately 8 mm medially from the junction of the middle and medial thirds of the cornea for medial surgery and 8 mm lateral from the junction of the middle and lateral third of the cornea for lateral surgery.

C   The limbal incision is made at the limbal fusion of conjunctiva and anterior Tenon's capsule for approximately 2 or 3 clock hours, and then two radial relaxing incisions are made through conjunctiva and anterior Tenon's capsule extending approximately 5 to 7 mm from the limbus.

D   1   The incision for exposure of the inferior oblique in the inferior-temporal quadrant
   2   The incision for exposure of the superior oblique between the superior rectus and trochlea
   3   The incision for exposure of the superior oblique at its insertion

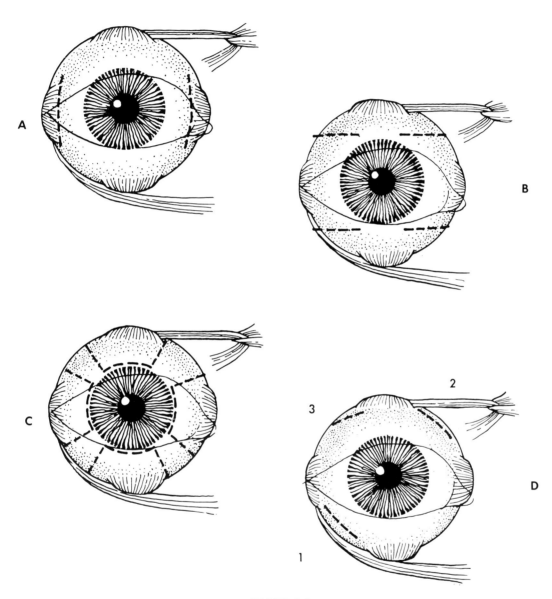

PLATE 4-1

THE SWAN TRANSCONJUNCTIVAL INCISION

PLATE 4-2

A The site of the incision for medial rectus surgery is approximately 6.5 mm from the limbus, 10 mm long, and concentric with the limbus. (For lateral rectus surgery the incision is made 7.9 mm from the limbus.)

B After the initial incision is made through the *conjunctiva only,* the conjunctiva is freed from anterior Tenon's capsule beneath for 5 mm or more, anterior and posterior to the conjunctival incision. The conjunctiva may be quite thin and friable, especially in adults.

C Anterior Tenon's capsule is picked up separately with fine-toothed forceps and a "buttonhole" incision is made through it. This anterior Tenon's capsule incision may be made at either the upper or lower border of the rectus muscle and is extended several millimeters along the long axis of the muscle (at right angles to the conjunctival incision). This incision exposes the muscle, which is still within its sheath. The muscle sheath and the intermuscular membrane that together comprise posterior Tenon's capsule are still intact.

D Two small muscle hooks are used to retract the edges of the incision that has been made in anterior Tenon's capsule. This exposes the muscle in its sheath more completely.

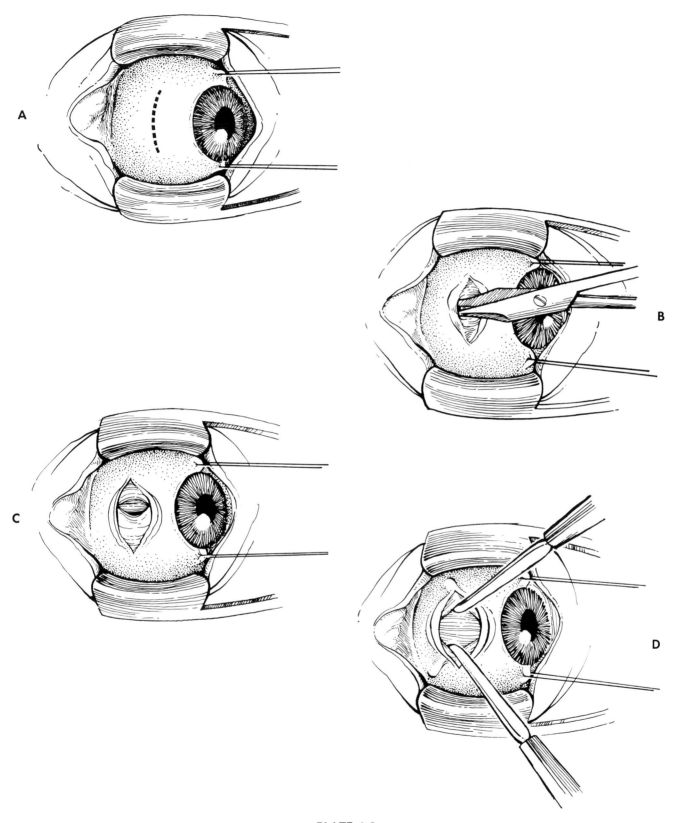

PLATE 4-2

43

THE SWAN TRANSCONJUNCTIVAL INCISION—cont'd

PLATE 4-3

A A small buttonhole incision has been made in the intermuscular membrane, exposing bare sclera, and a moderately sized right angle muscle hook has been placed behind the muscle and the tip exposed at the opposite border. After the rectus muscle has been engaged cleanly on the hook, recession, resection, myotomy, transfer, or advancement may be carried out by whatever technique the surgeon prefers. The extent to which intermuscular membrane is incised at the muscle's upper and lower border is determined by the surgeon.

B After surgery has been performed on the muscle, anterior Tenon's capsule is closed separately with one or two absorbable sutures tied with the knots buried.

C Conjunctiva is closed with several interrupted, fine absorbable sutures.

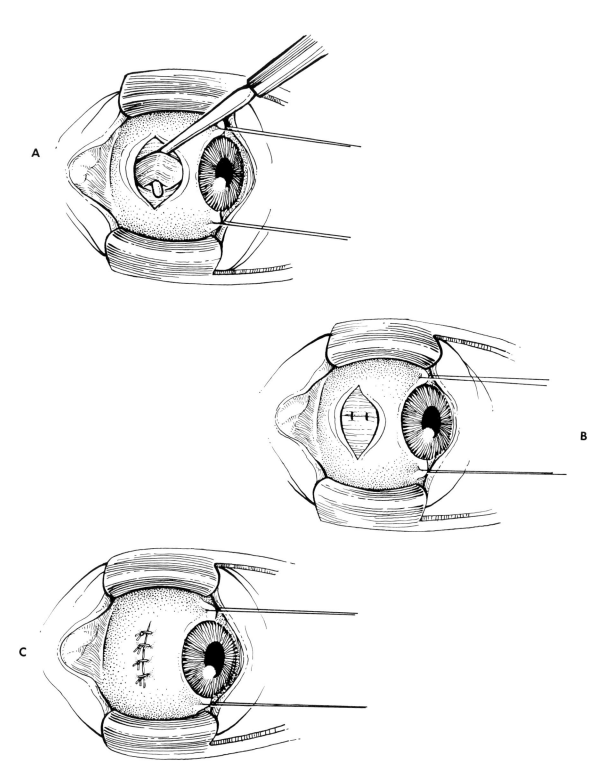

PLATE 4-3

THE CUL-DE-SAC INCISION (PARKS)

PLATE 4-4

A The incision for medial rectus surgery is made approximately 4.0 mm below the limbus. It extends 8 mm medially from the junction of the middle and medial thirds of the cornea, stopping just short of the base of the plica. A single snip incision through conjunctiva, anterior Tenon's capsule, and intermuscular membrane exposes bare sclera.

B The tip of a large muscle hook is placed upon bare sclera and the hook is guided upward along bare sclera until it is beneath the medial rectus muscle. The hook is then drawn toward the limbus to engage the muscle at its insertion.

C A second large muscle hook is placed *beneath* anterior Tenon's capsule and is guided superiorly over the original hook. The second hook is then moved back and forth over the first hook to free the fine attachments between anterior Tenon's capsule and the muscle sheath (during this maneuver the muscle in its sheath lies between the two hooks).

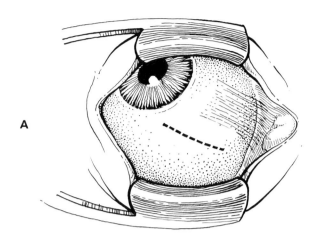

A

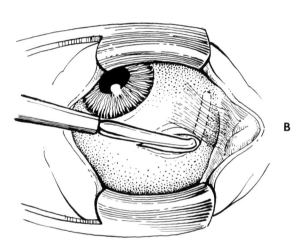

B

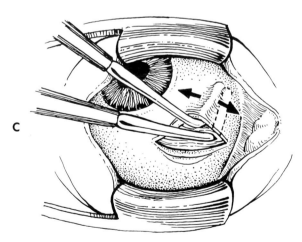

C

PLATE 4-4

PLATE 4-5

A The second muscle hook, having loosened the fascial connections between anterior Tenon's capsule and muscle sheath, is used to retract anterior Tenon's capsule and conjunctiva upward (superiorly), exposing the tip of the first muscle hook, which is now seen at the superior border of the muscle. A snip incision through the intermuscular membrane with scissors may be required to fenestrate the intermuscular membrane, exposing the tip of the first muscle hook. Intermuscular membrane is dissected from the muscle borders according to the surgeon's preference.

B With the muscle exposed, sutures may be placed for a recession procedure as shown. If a resection is to be done, an additional muscle hook or muscle clamp must be inserted to expose the tendon and muscle posteriorly.

C After suture placement for recession, the muscle has been severed from the globe. It is essential to use two fixation forceps, preferably of the self-locking type, at the corners of the insertion to stabilize the globe and to keep the incision centered over the operative site.

D At the conclusion of the procedure the conjunctiva and anterior Tenon's capsule are allowed to relax and "slide" back to the original incision site behind the lid. When properly done this procedure results in a very benign appearance of the eye in the immediate postoperative period because the incision is hidden by the lower lid.

An inferior incision may be closed with interrupted absorbable sutures or the incison may be left unsutured. A superior incision should always be closed because of the possibility of prolapsed Tenon's capsule hanging down in the palpebral space. This technique for exposure of the extraocular muscles is more difficult than the limbal or transconjunctival incision. The cul-de-sac incision does not allow for conjunctival recession and is not well suited for reoperations.

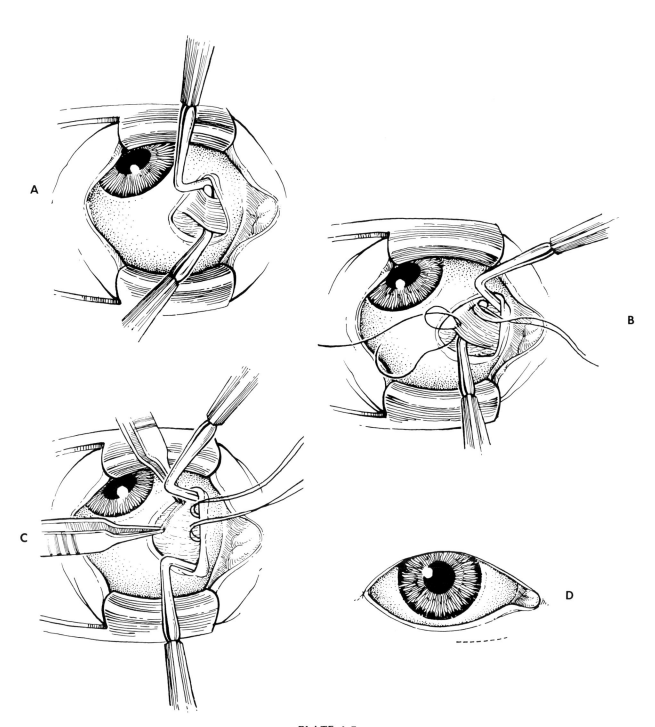

PLATE 4-5

THE LIMBAL INCISION

PLATE 4-6

A The site of the limbal incision for medial rectus surgery of the right eye is centered at the insertion of the medial rectus muscle and extends a total of 3 clock hours. The fusion of conjunctiva and anterior Tenon's capsule is grasped with fine-toothed forceps and tented up, and subanterior Tenon's space is entered with a No. 15 Bard-Parker blade (scissors may also be used as shown).

B Scissors are used to complete the limbal peritomy and two 5 to 7 mm radial relaxing incisions are made at the 1:30 and 4:30 o'clock meridians.

C Scissors and sharp dissection are used to sever the attachments between the muscle sheath and the undersurface of anterior Tenon's capsule. Bare sclera is exposed at each border of the muscle's insertion by piercing the intermuscular membrane at each edge of the muscle's insertion. It is imperative that bare sclera be identified during this maneuver. This is necessary for smooth passage of the muscle hook behind the insertion of the rectus muscle.

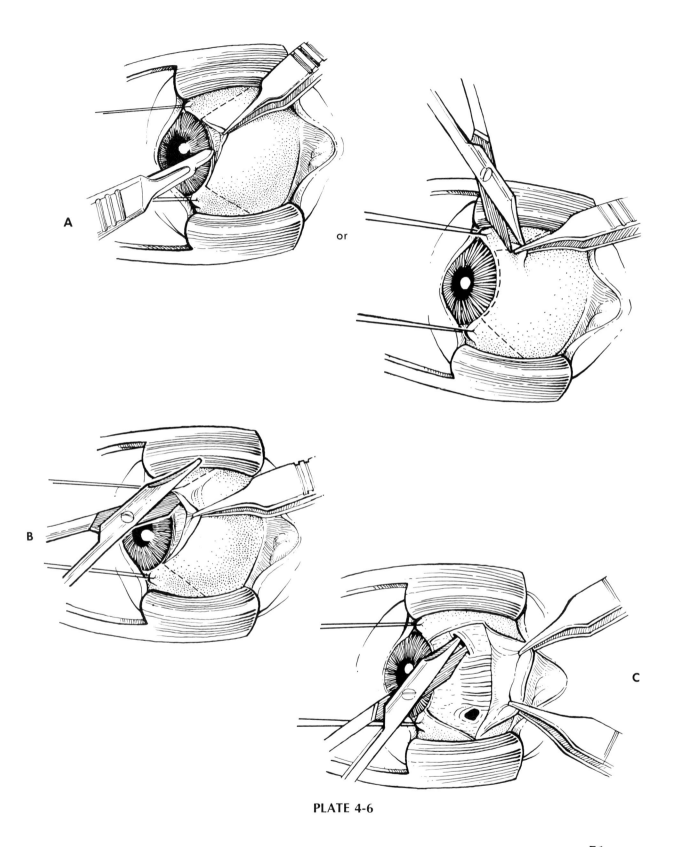

A

or

B

C

PLATE 4-6

51

THE LIMBAL INCISION—cont'd

PLATE 4-7

A When bare sclera is identified at each border of the muscle, a muscle hook is passed easily behind the insertion. The intermuscular membrane is dissected from the borders of the muscle and the attachments between muscle sheath and the undersurface of anterior Tenon's capsule are dissected according to the surgeon's preference. (See Chapters 5 and 6.)

B A medial rectus recession has been carried out.

C The limbal flap is closed at the apices with interrupted sutures. An additional suture may be placed in each of the radial incisions.

D The limbal flap may be recessed from 5.0 to 10.0 mm using three sutures. Two of the sutures join the tips of the flap with the base of the relaxing wing incision, and the third suture secures the center of the flap to the superficial sclera.

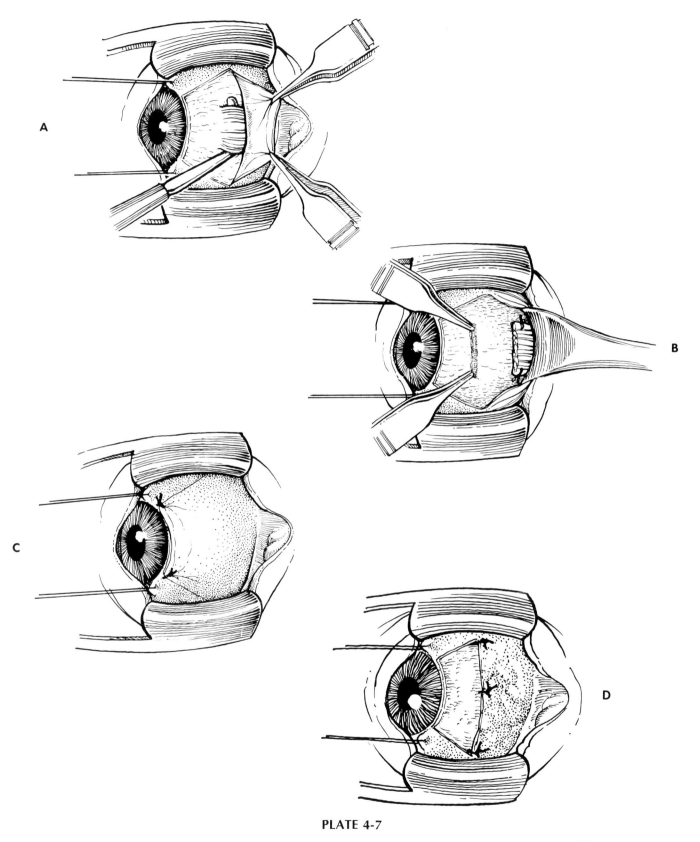

A

B

C

D

PLATE 4-7

OBLIQUE SURGERY INCISIONS

PLATE 4-8

A The incision for exposure of the superior oblique tendon medial to the superior rectus is begun at the medial aspect of the insertion of the superior rectus muscle (approximately 7.5 mm from the limbus) and extends through conjunctiva, anterior Tenon's capsule, and intermuscular membrane for 8.0 mm medially, concentric with the limbus.

B The incision for exposure of the superior oblique tendon at its insertion is begun at the lateral corner of the superior rectus insertion (approximately 8.5 mm from the limbus) and extends through conjunctiva, anterior Tenon's capsule, and intermuscular membrane laterally for 6.0 mm concentric with the limbus.

C The incision for exposure of the inferior oblique is made 9.0 mm from the limbus, is approximately 8.0 mm long, and is centered in the inferior temporal quadrant concentric with the limbus. The incision is carried through conjunctiva, anterior Tenon's capsule, and intermuscular membrane to bare sclera.

D The incision for a combined procedure on the lateral rectus and inferior oblique is a standard limbal incision that is extended 1 additional clock hour inferiorly.

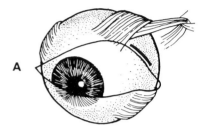

A

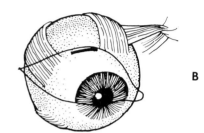

B

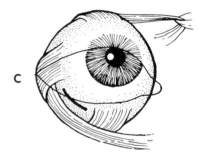

C

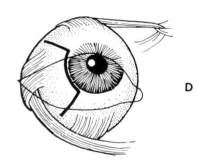

D

PLATE 4-8

CHAPTER FIVE

Recession technique of a rectus muscle

MEDIAL RECTUS RECESSION

Measured recession or retroplacement of the medial rectus is the procedure of choice for weakening this muscle in esodeviations. There are certain situations where marginal myotomy is a satisfactory and even preferred technique for weakening any of the rectus muscles, but marginal myotomies should be reserved for specific indications. (See Chapter 7.)

PLATE 5-1

A A minimum medial rectus recession is 2.5 mm. This is a reliable figure and should not be violated–that is, a medial rectus recession of less than 2.5 mm is never justified. The "resection effect" of suture placement and the fibrosis of healing tend to nullify any expected muscle weakening effect.

B A maximum medial rectus recession has traditionally been 5.5 mm. This figure is based on the fact that moving the medial rectus farther than 5.5 mm posterior to its normal insertion places the new insertion behind the point of tangency with the globe. This point of tangency is anterior to the equator of the globe because the origin of the medial rectus at the annulus of Zinn is medial to the anterior-posterior axis of the globe. If the contracting medial rectus acts upon the globe as if it were a string attached to a ball, no "unwrapping" or rotational effect would be expected if the muscle attached behind the point of tangency. The muscle in such an instance would act more as a retractor than an adductor. However, because medial rectus action on the globe is modified by attachments to the intermuscular membrane (posterior Tenon's capsule), certain cases requiring marked weakening of the medial rectus can be treated with a recession larger than 5.5 mm, or even with a free tenotomy in extreme cases. Because of variations in the point of insertion of the medial rectus (average 4.4 mm—range 3.0 to 6.0 mm) we now perform medial rectus recession using the limbus as the point of reference.

C It can be seen that even when the medial rectus is recessed to its functional point of tangency, attachments to the intermuscular membrane, which in turn attach to the globe well anterior to the point of tangency and medial to the globe's vertical axis, can mediate adduction. The lever arm is reduced but adducting power remains. The extent to which the intermuscular membrane is severed at the muscle border can influence the degree of weakening accomplished by a given medial rectus recession. An extreme example is the case of a slipped or "lost" muscle that has had extensive freeing of the intermuscular membrane from the muscle borders. In such a case, little if any adduction is present postoperatively. On the other hand, free tenotomy done with minimal dissection of the adjacent intermuscular membrane leaves the patient, in most cases, with some adduction. Free tenotomy is an unsound procedure more because it is unpredictable than because it is crippling.

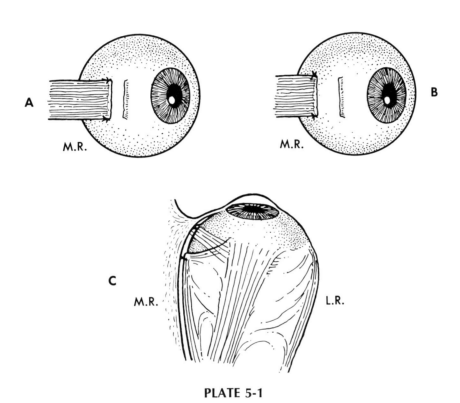

PLATE 5-1

LATERAL RECTUS RECESSION

Measured recession or retroplacement of the lateral rectus is the procedure of choice for weakening this muscle in exodeviations. In certain instances, a marginal myotomy is a satisfactory and even desirable procedure for weakening the lateral rectus muscle, but this procedure should be reserved for specific cases. (See Chapter 7.)

PLATE 5-2

A A minimum lateral rectus recession is 4.0 mm. Less recession should not be done if surgery to weaken the lateral rectus is justified in the first place.

B The maximum measured lateral rectus recession has customarily been 7.0 mm in adults and 6.0 mm in children. However, some surgeons perform 8.0-mm and even up to 10.0-mm recessions of the lateral rectus without a crippling of the muscle's effect. I personally have combined a double 80% marginal myotomy with an 8.0-mm recession of the lateral rectus in several cases where excess amounts of weakening of the lateral rectus were sought.

C The reason that large recessions of the lateral rectus may be done in certain cases without severely restricting motility is that the muscle continues to act through attachments to the intermuscular membrane. It can be seen that when the lateral rectus is recessed to its functional point of tangency, which is slightly behind the equator, it still influences globe movement by its attachments to the intermuscular membrane, which in turn attach anterior to the point of tangency. The lever arm is reduced but abducting power remains. The extent to which the intermuscular membrane is severed from the muscle border can influence the degree of weakening accomplished by a given lateral rectus recession. An extreme example is the case of a slipped or "lost" muscle that has had extensive freeing of the muscle borders from intermuscular membrane. In these cases, little if any abduction is present postoperatively. On the other hand, free tenotomy, which is always done with minimal dissection of the adjacent intermuscular membrane, in most cases leaves the patient with some abduction. Free tenotomy is an unsound procedure because it is unpredictable, not because it is crippling.

D When attempting to engage the lateral rectus with a muscle hook, care should be taken to avoid inadvertently including all or part of the inferior oblique muscle at its insertion. This complication can be avoided by making the initial sweep of the hook from above. If the hook is passed upward from below, it must not be thrust too deeply into the orbit. Inclusion of the inferior oblique in lateral rectus recession will produce excessive bleeding and, if undetected, can lead to unpredictable surgical results accompanied by restrictions in motility.

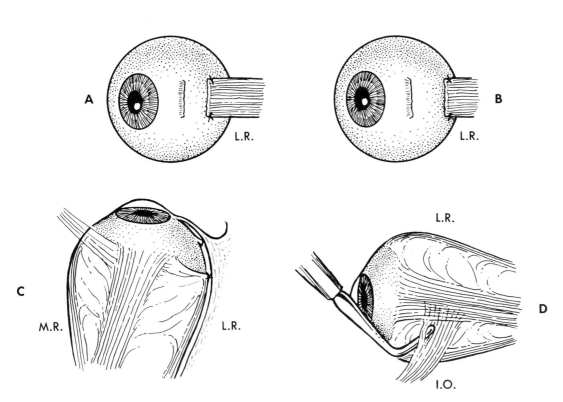

A

B L.R.

L.R.

C

M.R.

L.R.

L.R.

D

I.O.

PLATE 5-2

61

SUPERIOR RECTUS RECESSION

PLATE 5-3

A A minimum recession of the superior rectus is 2.5 mm. A recession smaller than this would be ineffective and should not be done.

B A maximum recession of the superior rectus is 5.0 mm although some surgeons exceed this figure. Large recessions of the superior rectus muscle do not cause retraction of the upper lid or objectionable widening of the palpebral fissure. The superior oblique tendon passes beneath the superior rectus approximately 5 mm posterior to the nasal aspect of the superior rectus insertion. A recession of the superior rectus greater than 5.0 mm would place the new insertion of the superior rectus at the superior oblique tendon.

C The superior rectus insertion can be engaged readily from the medial or the lateral side. Careful dissection exposing bare sclera should be completed before inserting the muscle hook.

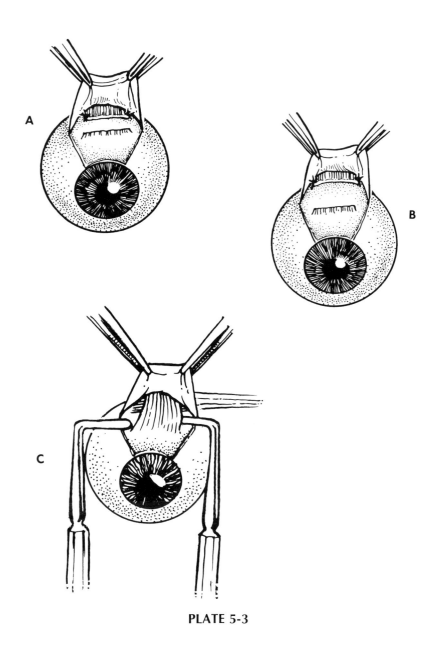

PLATE 5-3

63

INFERIOR RECTUS RECESSION

PLATE 5-4

A   A minimum recession of the inferior rectus is 2.5 mm. A recession smaller than this would be ineffective and should not be done.

B   A maximum recession of the inferior rectus under most circumstances is 5.0 mm. This figure is not ordinarily exceeded because an excessively large recession of the inferior rectus causes ptosis of the lower lid and a cosmetically objectionable widening of the palpebral fissure. This results from a downward and backward pull on the lower lid caused by the fact that the sheath of the inferior rectus is attached to Lockwood's ligament and the inferior oblique muscle, which in turn are attached to the inferior orbital septum and lower lid. Careful dissection of the intermuscular membrane of the inferior rectus and of the fascial attachments between the inferior rectus and Lockwood's ligament can minimize the effect of a large inferior rectus recession on the lower lid. It should be kept in mind that the nerve to the inferior oblique enters this muscle as it crosses the lateral border of the inferior rectus 12 mm posterior to the inferior rectus insertion. This nerve should be avoided when dissecting the inferior rectus. Inflammatory changes in the extraocular muscles associated with Graves' disease have a predilection for the inferior rectus. When these changes cause a hypotropia with restriction of forced elevation of the globe, the maximum figure for inferior rectus recession must be exceeded in order to obtain adequate elevation of the "bound down globe." In such a case, inferior rectus recession with an adjustable suture may be carried out.

C   When dissecting the inferior rectus in cases with or without restriction care should be taken to avoid cutting the vortex veins that lie at each border of the muscle between 8 and 12 mm behind the insertion. Also, Lockwood's ligament should be dissected carefully, using scissors with small snips under direct vision for a distance of 12 mm or slightly more posterior to the insertion. This technique reduces bleeding and reduces the likelihood of lower lid retraction with recession or advancement with resection.

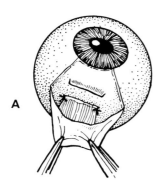

A

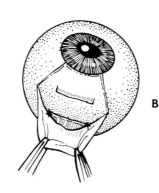

B

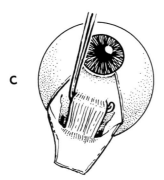

C

PLATE 5-4

RECTUS MUSCLE RECESSION TECHNIQUE

The standard technique for recession of each of the rectus muscles is the same. Differences in maximum and minimum amounts and management of the intermuscular membrane and check ligaments were discussed on preceding pages.

PLATE 5-5

A Exposure of the horizontal rectus is carried out by carefully incising the intermuscular membrane 2 or 3 mm from the muscle border with sharp dissection using scissors. The origin of anterior Tenon's capsule, which arises from the outer surface of the muscle sheath, is also severed with scissors. A severed band of what are ordinarily called check ligaments remains on the muscle's capsule. A small muscle hook may then be passed carefully over both the outer and the inner surface of the muscle to a point well behind the equator, ensuring that the muscle is free of attachments so that it may be retroplaced effectively.

B When the muscle is properly exposed, it is stabilized with a muscle hook, and a double loop is taken at each muscle border using a single arm suture of the surgeon's choice. The loops should include 2 or 3 mm of the muscle border and are placed approximately 0.5 to 1 mm from the tendinous insertion. The sutures are tied with a simple square knot, and the suture ends are tagged with a serrefine. The anterior ciliary vessels should be included in the double loop to aid in hemostasis when the muscle is cut from the globe.

C The muscle is then cut off *flush* with the sclera using scissors and taking *small* snips. Several foot plates may have to be severed before the muscle retracts freely.

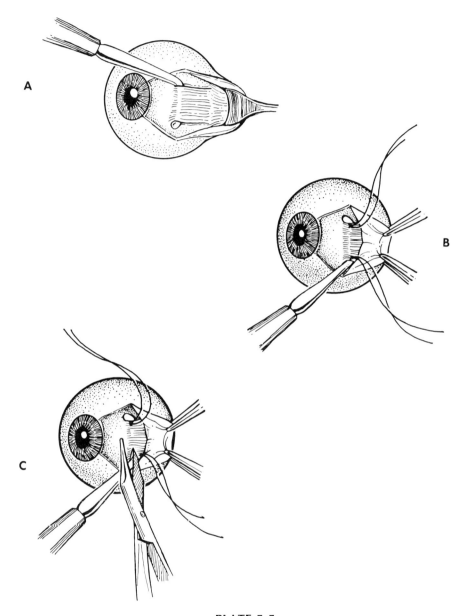

A

B

C

PLATE 5-5

RECTUS MUSCLE RECESSION TECHNIQUE—cont'd

Some surgeons prefer to recess a muscle using one double arm suture.

PLATE 5-7

A The suture is passed through the tendon, splitting it from side to side, and a locking loop is then taken at each border. The muscle is detached from the globe and an angled scleral bite is taken and the suture ends are tied.

B A single suture may be used, taking a bite into the central tendon, then additional bites are taken at the muscle borders and a locked loop is placed. The scleral bite is taken and the suture is brought through the original insertion and tied.

C The "crossed swords" technique of Parks may be used. The first needle is left in the scleral tunnel while the second needle is placed in sclera crossing the first. Both needles are brought out together. This maneuver is done to avoid the second needle cutting the first suture while in its scleral track.

D The figure-eight suture described by Reinecke is designed for use with fine (usually 6-0) nonabsorbable suture. Two-millimeter bites are taken in the sclera parallel to the insertion and the knot remains buried beneath the muscle so it is less likely to erode through conjunctiva. A Beren's muscle clamp must be used.

One of the main purposes for suturing the muscle to the globe in recession is to keep the muscle from slipping back, but these sutures also function to keep the muscle from *creeping forward!* For this reason a scleral bite should be taken at precisely the point where the muscle is to be anchored.

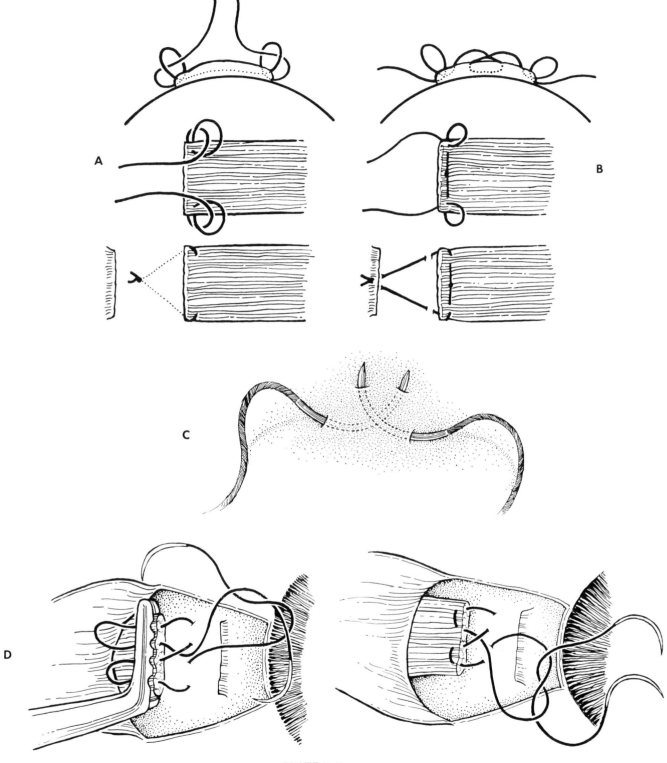

PLATE 5-7

VERTICAL DISPLACEMENT OF THE HORIZONTAL RECTUS

In cases of vertically incomitant strabismus (A or V pattern) without apparent overaction or underaction of the obliques, vertical displacement of the rectus muscles is effective in reducing or eliminating the vertical incomitance. The muscles are moved vertically to produce *more* or *less* relative strengthening or weakening in up or down gaze. For example, a horizontal rectus muscle that has been recessed or resected is relatively weakened in the field of action corresponding to the vertical direction in which its insertion has been moved. A resected medial rectus that has been moved downward receives relatively less strengthening effect in down gaze and relatively more strengthening effect in up gaze. A recessed medial rectus that is moved downward is excessively weakened in down gaze and minimally weakened in up gaze. The reason for this is that the distance between the new muscle attachment and the muscle's origin is reduced when the direction of gaze and the direction of the insertion shift coincide.

PLATE 5-8

A In order to know the proper direction for vertical displacement, the surgeon need only remember that the medial rectus muscles are *always* moved toward the "closed" end of the A or V and the lateral rectus muscles are *always* moved to the "open" end. It is taken for granted that the surgeon recesses the medial rectus for esodeviations and resects it for exodeviations. Likewise he recesses the lateral rectus for exodeviations and resects it for esodeviations.

B In A esotropia the medial rectus muscles are shifted upward. This may be done a minimum of 5.0 mm (approximately half the muscle width) to a maximum of 10.0 mm (approximately one muscle width). At the present it is not firmly established that graded amounts of vertical displacement result in graded amounts of A or V pattern reduction. In this type of recession it is important to place the new insertion concentric with the limbus. For this reason it is probably best to use calipers and measure from the limbus. In cases of A or V pattern without strabismus in the primary position, the horizontal rectus muscles may be shifted upward or downward with only enough recession to offset the resection effect of suture placement.

C In the case of a V esotropia the medial rectus muscles are recessed and shifted downward.

D In V exotropia the lateral rectus muscles are recessed and shifted upward.

E In A pattern exotropia the lateral rectus muscles are recessed and shifted downward.

F Vertical shifting of the horizontal rectus may be carried out when a recession-resection procedure is done. The same rules apply. In the example shown a recession-resection has been done for an A pattern exotropia. The left medial rectus has been resected as it should be for an exodeviation and it has been moved upward toward the "closed" end of the A. The lateral rectus has been recessed as it should be for an exodeviation and it has been moved downward toward the "open" end of the A.

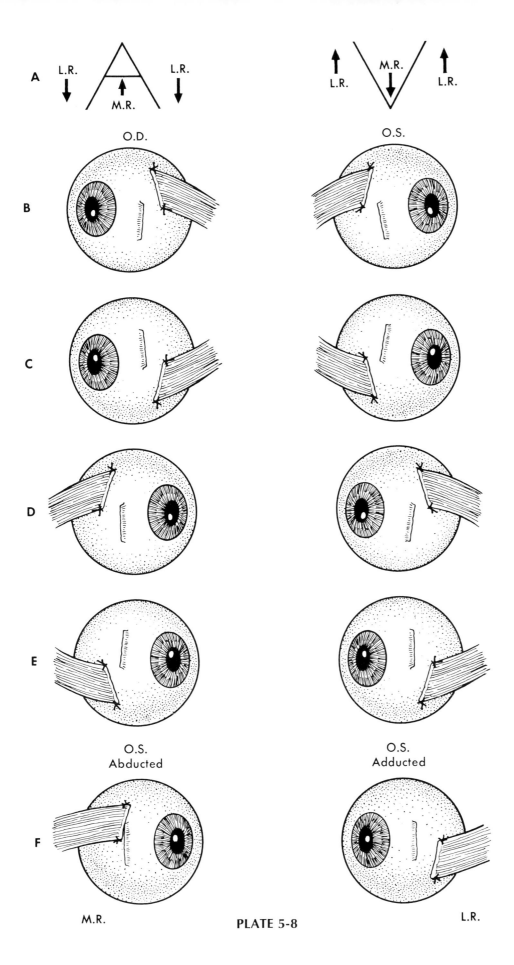

A
L.R. M.R. L.R.
L.R. M.R. L.R.

O.D.   O.S.

B

C

D

E

O.S.
Abducted

O.S.
Adducted

F

M.R.   PLATE 5-8   L.R.   73

Horizontal displacement of the vertical rectus muscles has been suggested by Miller.

The superior rectus muscles are moved nasally to "close" a V pattern or temporally to "open" an A pattern. The inferior rectus muscles are moved medially to "close" an A pattern or temporally to "open" a V pattern. Horizontal displacement of the vertical rectus is seldom done.

CHAPTER SIX

Resection technique of a rectus muscle

Resection of an extraocular muscle is generally classified as a "strengthening" procedure. Of course, removal of all or part of a muscle's tendon with or without some muscle fibers merely shortens and does not strengthen a muscle, at least after the initial reflex spasticity subsides. Some surgeons have stated that the principal beneficial effect of a resection is to enhance the effect of a recession procedure done on the antagonist. As I am becoming more aware of the relationship between passive mechanical factors and dynamic neural factors in the surgical management of strabismus, I find myself doing fewer resections.

HORIZONTAL RECTUS RESECTION (MEDIAL AND LATERAL RECTUS MUSCLES)

PLATE 6-1

A The minimum amount for resection for either a medial rectus or a lateral rectus muscle is 5.0 mm, regardless of the age of the patient. In general, a resection procedure done on a horizontal rectus muscle is less effective in terms of altering ocular alignment than a recession procedure of the same amount, hence the larger relative minimal values for horizontal rectus resection.

B The maximum resection for a horizontal rectus muscle is 8.0 mm for infants under age 1 year and is ordinarily 10.0 mm for older children and adults. However, upper limit figures for resection procedures are very loosely adhered to, in contrast to the minimum figures for horizontal rectus resections, which should not be violated. In a patient with a very large deviation, horizontal rectus resection of up to 14.0 mm may be done. Some incomitance may result in these cases but the benefits accrued far outweigh the undesirable consequences of incomitance. For example, a blind eye with 90 Δ of exotropia occurring in a patient who wishes no extraocular muscle surgery on the seeing eye can be treated with a large (up to 14.0 mm) resection of the medial rectus and a large recession of the lateral rectus, perhaps combined with a marginal myotomy. This will result in straighter eyes in the primary position, and, in my experience, the incomitance produced is not bothersome to the patient and is not a cosmetic defect. Many more problems are created by horizontal resections that are too small than by those that are too large.

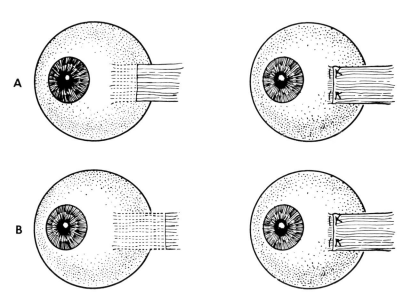

PLATE 6-1

MANAGEMENT OF THE CHECK LIGAMENTS AND INTERMUSCULAR MEMBRANE IN HORIZONTAL RECTUS RESECTION

PLATE 6-2

A When first exposed prior to resection, a horizontal rectus muscle is found encased within its sheath, which is continuous with the intermuscular membrane (posterior Tenon's capsule). "Inner check ligaments" also connect the anterior muscle sheath to the inner aspect of anterior Tenon's capsule. At this point in surgery the question arises: is horizontal rectus resection more effective and/or more predictable when a minimal dissection of the intramuscular membrane is done or when a maximum dissection of the intermuscular membrane is done?

B Prior to placement of the muscle clamp, the decision is made to carry out either extensive or minimal dissection of the intermuscular membrane and check ligaments.

C The intermuscular membrane is dissected from the muscle borders to a point just behind the line of insertion of the resection clamp if minimal intermuscular membrane and check ligament dissection is elected. The resection is then carried out in the usual manner.

D When the resection is completed, intermuscular membrane is adjacent to the muscle insertion.

E The intermuscular membrane and overlying "internal" check ligaments are severed to a point well behind the equator if maximum intermuscular membrane and check ligament dissection is elected. This means that when the muscle clamp is placed across the muscle at the intended point of resection, several millimeters of muscle border have been dissected free from the intermuscular membrane posterior to the clamp's position.

F When the resection is completed, the intermuscular membrane is several millimeters behind the point of reinsertion.

Fifty consecutive horizontal rectus resections were done using minimal and maximal dissection techniques alternately. It was found that a slightly greater effect and slightly more predictable resection results were obtained after maximal dissection of the intermuscular membrane. This is contrary to a popularly held belief that leaving as much of the intermuscular membrane as possible intact causes greater effect from horizontal rectus resection. In addition, minimum check ligament dissection can produce undesirable limited ductions in the field of action of the resected muscle because of the anterior displacement of the internal check ligaments.

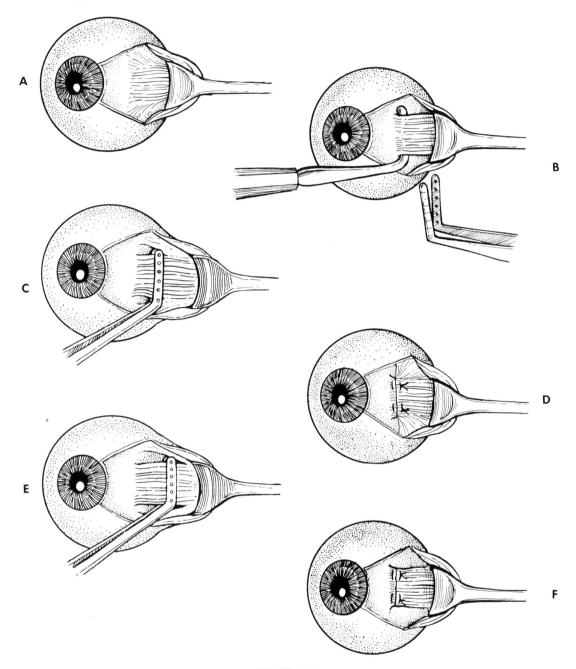

PLATE 6-2

79

RESECTION CLAMP TECHNIQUE FOR RECTUS MUSCLE RESECTION

The technique for resection of the medial and lateral rectus is identical.

PLATE 6-3

A   The muscle is exposed and the intermuscular membrane and check ligaments are dissected according to the surgeon's preference. A muscle clamp
is placed across the muscle to include the amount of muscle and tendon
the surgeon intends to resect. A caliper is used to measure from the muscle
hook, which is behind the insertion of the muscle to the anterior edge of
the clamp. Necessary adjustments in the position of the clamp are made.
The muscle should not be stretched at this time. Some surgeons prefer to
measure from a point just anterior to the muscle hook, which is behind the
insertion to a point just posterior to the muscle clamp, the point where the
sutures are eventually placed. Larger "numbers" will result when this type
measurement is done but the same size resection will obviously be accomplished. The most important thing to remember in measuring a resection or any extraocular muscle strengthening or weakening procedure is
that consistency in technique on the part of the surgeon is the only way to
achieve predictable results. Because of such opportunities for variations in
technique, one surgeon's numbers do not transfer to another.

B   The tendon is severed from its insertion. A 1-mm tendinous stump should
be left at the insertion to serve as an anchoring place for sutures. The sclera
immediately behind the insertion of the rectus muscles is only 0.3 mm
thick, so this tendinous stump provides a safety factor during suture placement.

C   Double arm sutures are inserted in a backhand manner through the tendinous insertion.

D   They are carried through the muscle behind or posterior to the resection
clamp. The assistant grasps the needle tip and pulls the suture through.

E   The two double arm sutures are shown after having been placed in a horizontal mattress fashion, first through the insertion and then through the
muscle behind the clamp.

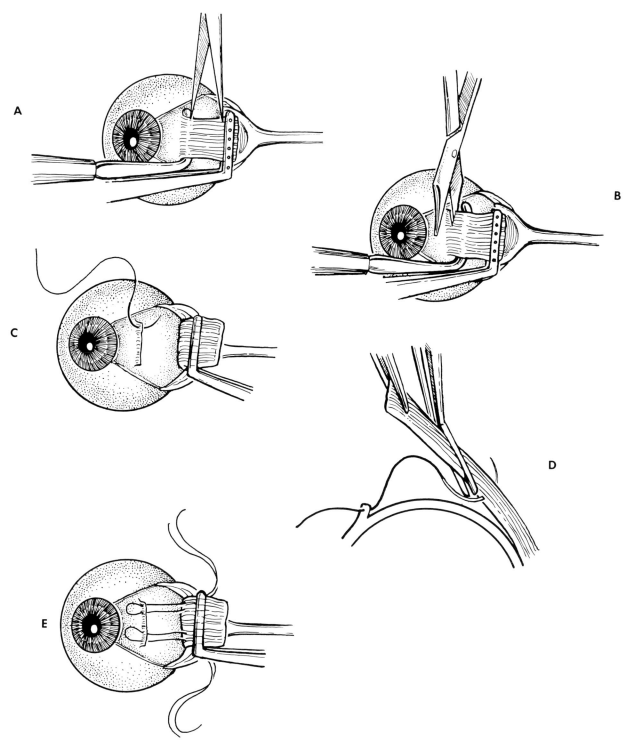

PLATE 6-3

RESECTION CLAMP TECHNIQUE FOR RECTUS MUSCLE RESECTION—cont'd

PLATE 6-4

A The resection clamp is moved to the tip of the tendon. A Nugent forceps is used to hold the tip of the tendon while the resection clamp is advanced.

B Traction is placed on the muscle clamp to advance the muscle so that the point of passage of the sutures through the muscle is directly over the line of the original muscle insertion. The sutures are tied securely with a surgeon's knot.

C A hemostat is used to crush the tendon just anterior to the point where the sutures are tied in an effort to control bleeding.

D Scissors are used to excise the excess tendon.

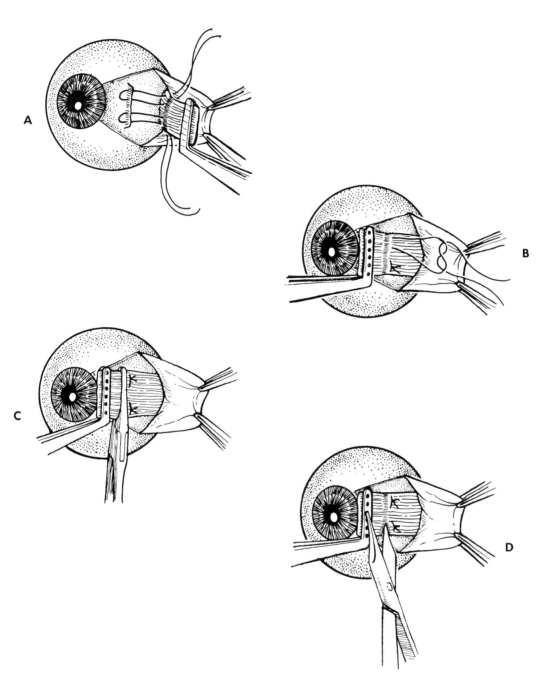

PLATE 6-4

RESECTION CLAMP TECHNIQUE FOR RECTUS MUSCLE RESECTION—cont'd

PLATE 6-5

A With the excess tendon removed, the resected muscle abuts the point of the original tendinous insertion. The double horizontal mattress sutures with bites several millimeters apart afford a secure reunion of the resected muscle across its entire width.

B A cross section at the point of union shows that the tendon stump and muscle are joined in a slightly puckered out butt joint. This gradually smooths down over several weeks, producing a smooth appearance to conjunctiva overlying the resected muscle insertion.

C Sutures may be placed through the stump of the muscle from the muscle side.

D A lap joint is produced when sutures are so placed.

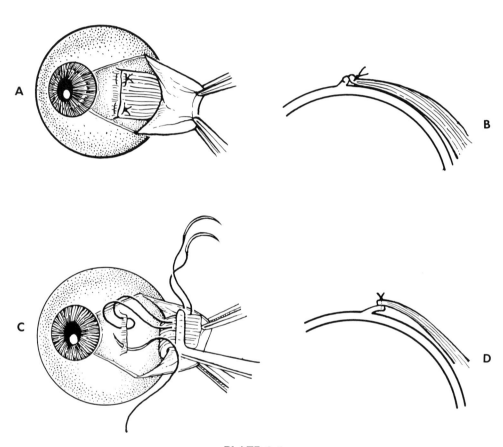

PLATE 6-5

DOUBLE ARM SUTURE TECHNIQUE FOR RECTUS MUSCLE RESECTION

Some surgeons prefer to resect the rectus muscles, either horizontal or vertical, using one double arm suture. This technique lacks some of the "insurance" factors of using two separate horizontal mattress sutures, but according to those surgeons who prefer this technique, it is completely safe.

PLATE 6-6

A The muscle is exposed and, after measurement, the extent of tendon and muscle resection is determined. A suture, usually 4-0 or 5-0, or possibly 6-0 if a synthetic absorbable suture is used, splits the muscle at this point from edge to edge. A 3.0-mm loop is then taken slightly behind this suture line at each muscle border and the loops are locked.

B An "on end" view of this suture placement is shown here.

C The section of the muscle to be resected is excised with scissors after the muscle is crushed just behind the insertion and just in front of the suture line with a hemostat. Each arm of the suture is brought out through the edge of the stump of the muscle's original insertion.

D Each suture is then brought back through the insertion near its center. The sutures are brought through the central portion of the muscle from beneath. The suture is gently "sawed" to bring the remaining muscle up to the original insertion.

E A surgeon's knot is tied, securing the resected muscle in place.

F A figure-eight suture can be used for rectus muscle resection. When such a resection technique is done, the Beren's clamp (Plate 5-7, D) is first placed on the muscle according to the amount of intended resection, the segment of muscle is resected, and the suture is placed and tied as diagrammed. The resected muscle is anchored just anterior at the muscle's original insertion with 2.0-mm scleral bites.

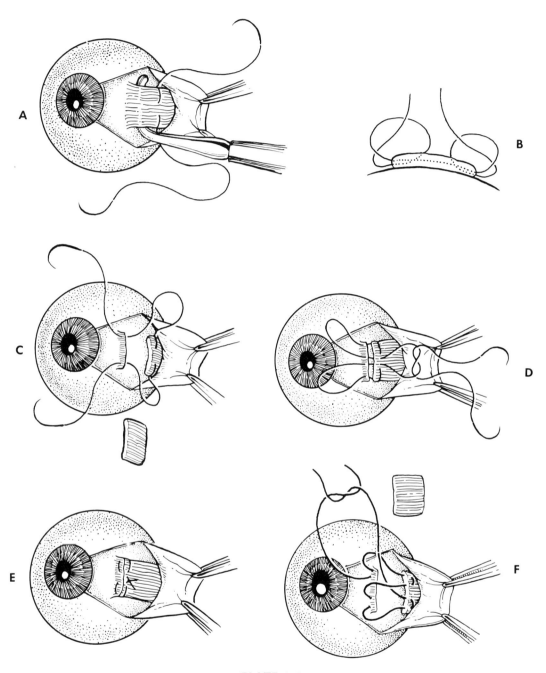

PLATE 6-6

RESECTION OF THE SUPERIOR RECTUS

The minimum superior rectus resection is 2.5 to 3.0 mm and the maximum is 5.0 mm. Resection of less than 2.5 to 3.0 mm is probably ineffective, and resection of more than 5.0 mm causes a forward and downward shift of the upper lid, creating ptosis.

Because of the proximity of the superior oblique tendon to the insertion of the superior rectus, dissection of the intermuscular membrane of the superior rectus prior to resection must be done carefully. This dissection should be carried back only a millimeter or so beyond the extent of the intended resection. The limited room available in the area of the superior rectus makes a free suture technique for resection preferable to the muscle clamp technique used for horizontal rectus resection.

PLATE 6-7

A After exposure of the muscle, a 3.0-mm double loop suture is placed at each muscle border at the intended point of resection. These sutures are tied with square knots and should ligate the anterior ciliary vessels.

B A hemostat is used to crush the tendon just anterior to the point of suture placement.

C Scissors sever the tendon just anterior to the point of suture placement.

D The tendon is trimmed from its insertion, leaving a 1.0-mm stump.

E The previously placed sutures are used to reattach the tendon to the stump of the muscle at the point of the original insertion. Very frequently a gap exists in the center of the muscle.

F A third suture placed at the center of the insertion eliminates the gapping and provides a more secure reunion of the muscle and insertion.

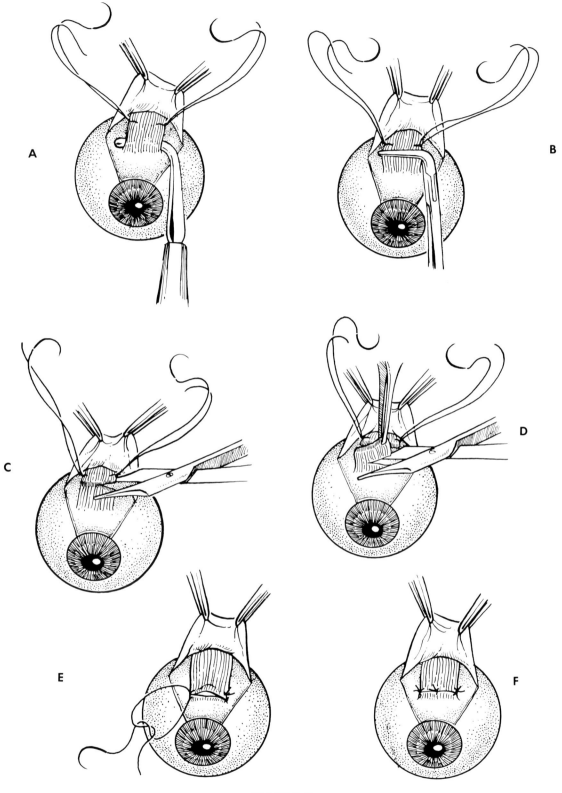

PLATE 6-7

INFERIOR RECTUS RESECTION TECHNIQUE

The minimum inferior rectus resection is 2.5 to 3.0 mm and the maximum is 5.0 mm, under ordinary circumstances. However, when a very large hyperdeviation is present, the surgeon may in some instances safely resect up to 9.0 mm or even more of the inferior rectus. The inferior rectus must be dissected carefully from its attachments to Lockwood's ligament, and care must be exercised to avoid damage to the inferior oblique nerve or muscle. Also, between 8.0 and 12.0 mm posterior to the inferior rectus insertion a vortex vein pierces sclera adjacent to the inferior rectus muscle's borders. Great care should be exercised to avoid cutting this vein (see Plate 5-4, C).

PLATE 6-8

A   In order to expose more of the inferior rectus muscle when a large resection is intended, two muscle hooks are used to expose the area of the resected muscle and tendon prior to placement of the sutures.

B   After measurement with calipers 3.0-mm double loop sutures are placed at the borders of the muscle. These sutures are then tied with a square knot. The anterior ciliary vessels should be ligated with this suture.

C   The muscle is clamped just anterior to the line of suture.

D   The tendon and muscle to be resected are excised using scissors.

E   The two sutures are used to reattach the tendon to the original insertion, and usually a third central suture is required to prevent gapping in the center.

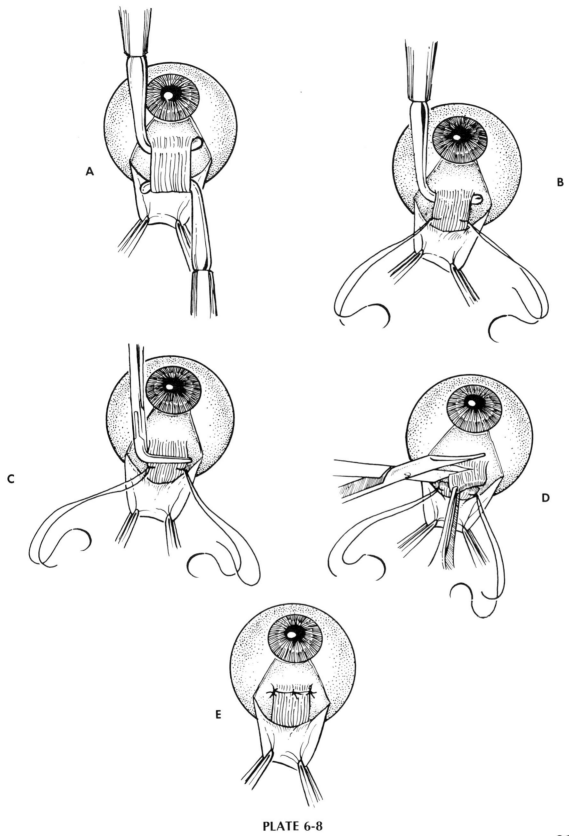

PLATE 6-8

DISPLACEMENT OF THE HORIZONTAL RECTUS MUSCLES WITH RESECTION FOR A AND V PATTERNS

PLATE 6-9

A A recession-resection procedure is carried out on the left eye of a patient with a V pattern exotropia. The resected left medial rectus is shifted a half muscle width downward, the recessed left lateral rectus is shifted a half muscle width upward.

B A recession-resection procedure of the right eye in a patient with an A exotropia is illustrated. The resected right medial rectus is shifted a half muscle width upward, the recessed right lateral rectus is shifted a half muscle width downward.

C In a bilateral lateral rectus resection procedure for an A pattern esotropia, both resected lateral rectus muscles are shifted one full muscle width downward.

D In a bilateral lateral rectus resection procedure for V pattern esotropia, both resected lateral rectus muscles are shifted one full muscle width upward.

As with all vertical displacements of the horizontal rectus, for treatment of vertically incomitant strabismus the lateral rectus muscles are moved toward the "open end" of the pattern and the medial rectus muscles are moved toward the "closed end" of the pattern. One need only remember that medial rectus muscles are weakened for esodeviation and the lateral rectus muscles are strengthened for esodeviations; conversely, the medial rectus muscles are strengthened and the lateral rectus muscles weakened for exodeviations.

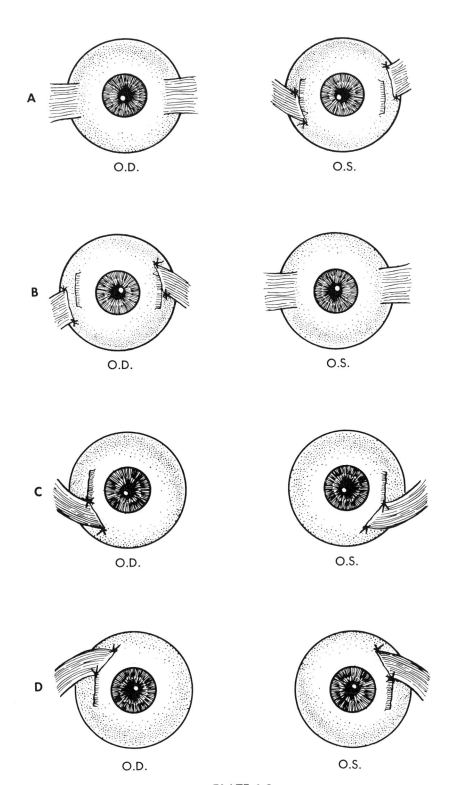

A

O.D.   O.S.

B

O.D.   O.S.

C

O.D.   O.S.

D

O.D.   O.S.

PLATE 6-9

CHAPTER SEVEN

Surgery of the obliques

The superior oblique is the muscle most frequently involved in acquired isolated extraocular muscle palsy, and oblique muscle surgery is usually indicated in persistent paretic cases because of a nonfusable torsional ocular misalignment with or without head tilt. In 130 patients with superior oblique palsy treated in our clinic over approximately a 6-year period, 104 required surgery on either the paretic superior oblique, the antagonist inferior oblique, or both. The diagnostic techniques and judgments associated with oblique muscle dysfunction may be considered by some to be challenging, but the surgical approach is actually straightforward.

WEAKENING THE INFERIOR OBLIQUE
Inferior oblique myectomy

PLATE 7-1

A   The incision for exposure of the inferior oblique muscle is approximately 8 mm long. It is located 9 mm from and is concentric with the limbus, and must be anterior to the inferior fat pad. Two fine-toothed forceps are used initially to elevate the conjunctiva, Tenon's capsule, and intermuscular membrane, and a snip incision is made between the forceps, exposing bare sclera. This snip incision is then enlarged to the full extent of 8.0 mm.

B   Blunt-tipped Wescott scissors are inserted into the incision against bare sclera and the scissors tips are spread to separate the filamentous attachments between sclera and the scleral surface of the inferior oblique muscle.

C   To engage the inferior oblique muscle under direct vision, the surgeon places a large muscle hook behind the insertion of the lateral and the inferior rectus muscles. A third muscle hook or a forcep is used to elevate the posterior tip of the conjunctiva–Tenon's incision. Deep in the incision at the junction of the sclera and posterior Tenon's capsule, the anterior border of the inferior oblique will be seen.

D   The anterior border of the inferior oblique is engaged first on a Steven's muscle hook. The surgeon must take great care to hook only the muscle and avoid fenestrating the intermuscular membrane (posterior Tenon's capsule), which would allow an undesirable prolapse of orbital fat that in turn could cause hemorrhage and postoperative restrictions.

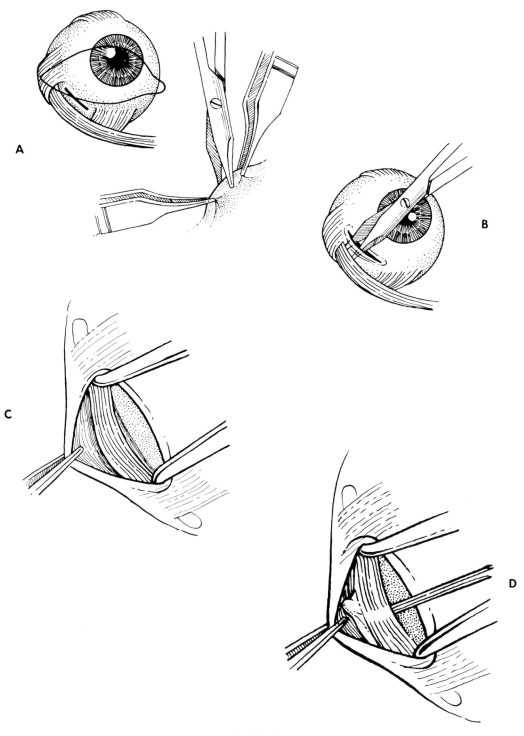

PLATE 7-1

PLATE 7-2

A Scissors or a scalpel blade are used to cut down on the tip of the Steven's hook, exposing it.

B The Steven's hook is replaced by two larger hooks, and the fascial layers associated with the muscle are dissected from the muscle, exposing 5 to 8 mm of the inferior oblique. (The muscle hooks behind the insertions of the lateral and inferior rectus muscles may be removed as soon as the large hooks are placed under the inferior oblique.)

C Two hemostats placed 5 to 8 mm apart are used to clamp the inferior oblique muscle belly.

D With scissors or a scalpel blade, a 5- to 8-mm segment of the belly of the inferior oblique muscle lying between the hemostats is excised. Cautery is then applied heavily to each cut end for hemostasis.

E After the hemostats are removed, the inferior oblique muscle is allowed to retract* and the conjunctival incision is closed with either interrupted or running sutures. This incision may also be left unsutured according to the surgeon's preference.

---

*Dunlap states that the globe should be rotated upward and inward at the conclusion of inferior oblique weakening to produce more consistent effects from such surgery.

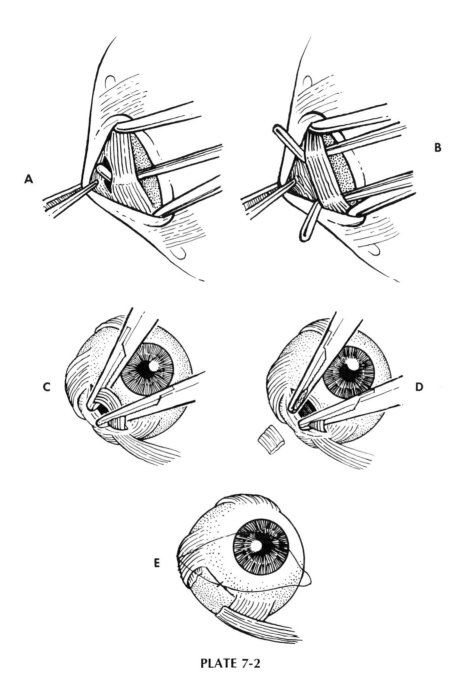

PLATE 7-2

WEAKENING THE INFERIOR OBLIQUE—cont'd
A common complication of inferior oblique weakening and how to avoid it

PLATE 7-3

A As is the case with any of the extraocular muscles, the function of the inferior oblique depends upon its having contractible tissue connecting the origin and insertion. By means of isotonic contraction these two points are brought closer together and the muscle's effect is manifested through movement of the globe toward the fixed point or origin of the muscle.

B If in the process of performing a myectomy or any weakening procedure of the inferior oblique muscle the muscle clamps or recession sutures include only a portion of the muscle (or to say it another way, exclude a portion of the muscle), a band of uninterrupted muscle tissue with associated intermuscular membrane remains connecting origin and insertion.

C A portion of the inferior oblique coursing uninterrupted between origin and insertion acts somewhat like a tendon. Isotonic contraction in such a case continues to have nearly the same effect as with the unoperated muscle.

D This complication, which causes undercorrections, can be avoided. Careful inspection of the posterior aspect of the inferior oblique muscle reveals any remaining bands. These are engaged on Steven's muscle hooks and a myectomy is repeated on this smaller segment of the inferior oblique muscle.

E In order for an inferior oblique myectomy to be effective, a segment of inferior oblique that includes its *entire* width must be removed. A partial myotomy of the inferior oblique is ineffective. When disinsertion of the inferior oblique is chosen for weakening this muscle, care must be taken to sever the entire insertion.

F Exclusion of a slip of the inferior oblique can be avoided before the myectomy is done if the posterior border of the inferior oblique is identified. As shown from the surgeon's view on a left inferior oblique muscle a slip has been missed in the initial hook placement.

G An additional hook has been placed behind the missed posterior slip of the inferior oblique.

H The two large hooks are replaced to include the entire inferior oblique muscle, and the inferior oblique muscle is ready for myectomy.

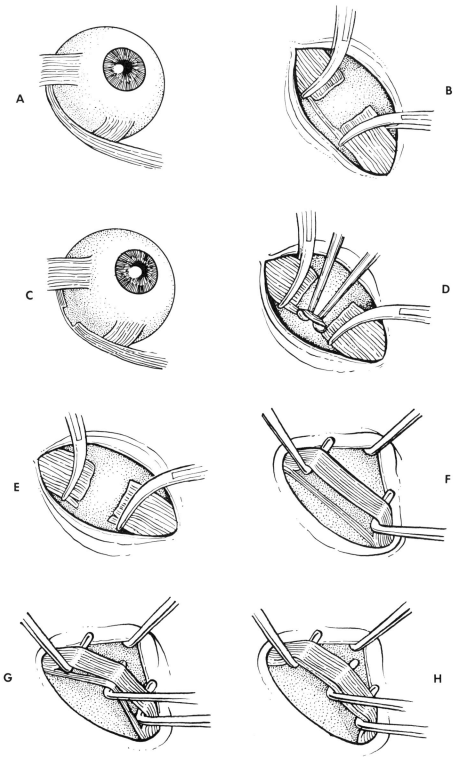

PLATE 7-3

WEAKENING THE INFERIOR OBLIQUE—cont'd
Alternative weakening procedures of the inferior oblique:
recession and disinsertion

PLATE 7-4

A The incision, localization, and exposure for recession or disinsertion of the inferior oblique muscle is the same as described previously for a myectomy.

B Recession of the inferior oblique muscle is begun by placing either two single arm sutures or a single double arm suture through the inferior oblique muscle near the lower border of the lateral rectus. The suture is therefore inserted several millimeters from the muscle's broad insertion. To ensure inclusion of all of the muscle fibers at this point, careful inspection should be carried out. The surgeon must inspect and detach the entire width of the inferior oblique muscle, freeing the muscle completely from the sclera.

C The inferior oblique is reattached to sclera at a point depending upon the amount of recession desired. Fink described an instrument for locating the point of reinsertion, but recession is now usually accomplished by reattaching the inferior oblique in relation to existing landmarks. Parks reattaches the anterior corner of the inferior oblique 2 mm lateral and 3 mm posterior to the lateral border of the inferior rectus insertion. The posterior scleral reattachment is placed according to the width of the inferior oblique muscle. Other techniques reinsert the inferior oblique slightly more posteriorly. The point of reattachment described by Parks is considerably anterior to the normal course of the inferior oblique muscle as it passes beneath the inferior rectus muscle. This should cause the recessed inferior oblique to become relatively more effective as an intorter and less effective as an elevator. This does not occur, possibly because the new effective insertion of the inferior oblique coincides with its normal attachment to Lockwood's ligament.

D Another technique for weakening the inferior oblique is disinsertion, as described by Dyer. In this procedure the insertion of the inferior oblique is exposed and the muscle is simply detached from the sclera. The muscle is allowed to retract and the incision is closed.

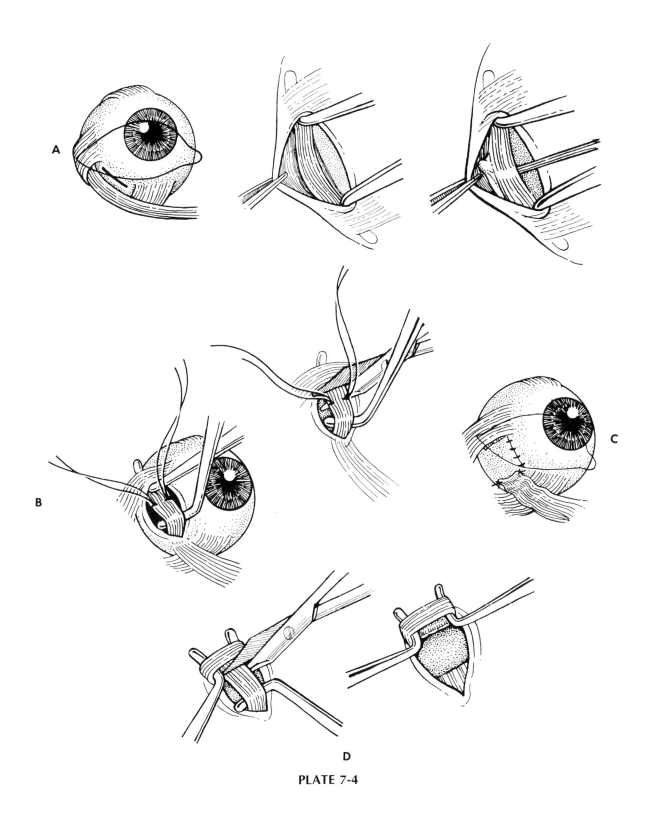

A

B

C

D

PLATE 7-4

STRENGTHENING THE INFERIOR OBLIQUE
Inferior oblique tuck: resection and advancement of the inferior oblique

Strengthening procedures done on the inferior oblique are the least effective of any surgery done on the vertically acting muscles and are rarely indicated. Two techniques for strengthening the inferior oblique–tuck and resection with advancement–have been described and will be illustrated.

PLATE 7-5

A To tuck the inferior oblique, the muscle is first localized and engaged in the inferior temporal quadrant exactly as is done prior to performing a myectomy. A tuck is then made in the muscle using a Fink tucker or a freehand technique. Nonabsorbable sutures such as 5-0 Merseline are used. When a tuck is done, no less than a total of 10.0 mm of the muscle should be included.

B In resection and advancement of the inferior oblique, two single arm sutures are placed at the borders of the inferior oblique muscle just below the inferior border of the lateral rectus. The sutures are therefore placed approximately 5.0 mm from the insertion.

C The muscle is clamped with a hemostat and is severed just distal to these sutures. The stump of the muscle is cut free from the globe at the insertion and is discarded.

D The inferior oblique is reattached to sclera at the upper border of the lateral rectus. The anterior suture is placed 12.0 mm posterior to the lateral rectus insertion and the posterior suture is placed slightly more posterior.

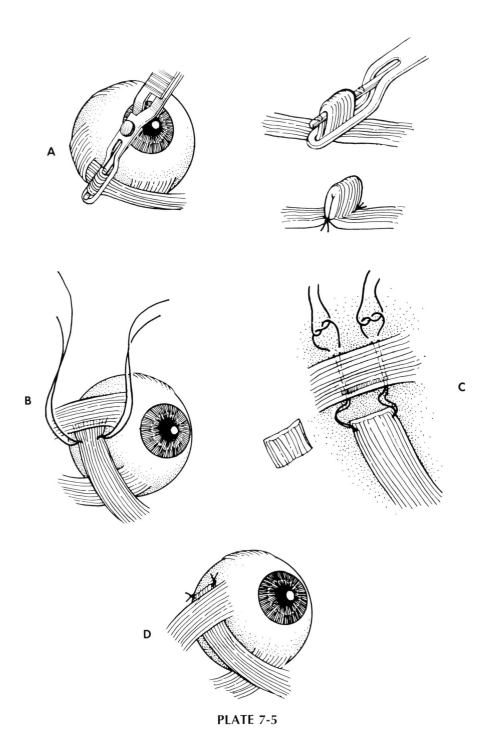

PLATE 7-5

WEAKENING PROCEDURES OF THE SUPERIOR OBLIQUE
Superior oblique tenotomy

The superior oblique is effectively weakened by a tenectomy, tenotomy, or recession. This should be done with minimal disruption of the tendon sheath and associated fascial layers.

PLATE 7-6

A The incision for exposure of the superior oblique tendon medial to the superior rectus is begun at the medial aspect of the insertion of the superior rectus muscle and extends through conjunctiva, anterior Tenon's capsule, and intermuscular membrane 8 mm medially and is concentric with the limbus.

B When bare sclera is exposed a moderate size muscle hook is placed behind the insertion of the superior rectus and the medial rectus, and a third muscle hook is placed beneath the free edge of the incision to retract intermuscular membrane, anterior Tenon's capsule, and conjunctiva. These three muscle hooks are held under slight tension to produce an incision the shape of an equilateral triangle. The surgeon then peers into the depths of the wound, observing the undersurface of anterior Tenon's capsule. A whitish band will be seen representing the superior oblique tendon within its sheath. The width of the superior oblique tendon at this point is approximately 3 mm.

C A Steven's or Hardesty hook is placed into the depths of the incision to engage the superior oblique tendon with a minimum of associated Tenon's capsule and intermuscular membrane.

D The tip of the Steven's hook is dissected free with scissors or a scalpel blade so that it projects cleanly behind the posterior aspect of the superior oblique tendon.

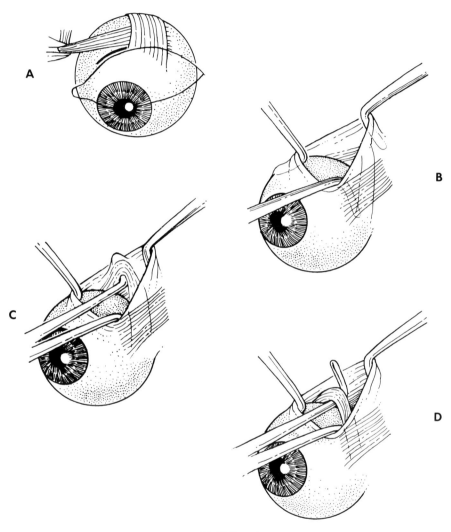

PLATE 7-6

SUPERIOR OBLIQUE TENOTOMY AFTER A TEMPORAL APPROACH

An alternative method for performing tenotomy of the superior oblique employs exposure of the superior oblique tendon at its insertion in a manner similar to the exposure for a superior oblique tuck at its insertion. The superior oblique tendon may be found readily. It is located approximately 6 to 12 mm posterior to the lateral corner of the insertion of the superior rectus, approximately at the lateral margin of the superior rectus.

PLATE 7-8

A The superior rectus tendon is engaged with a large muscle hook. A second muscle hook elevates the superior rectus muscle approximately 5 to 8 mm posterior to its insertion, and a third muscle hook retracts conjunctiva and anterior Tenon's capsule laterally and backward. The insertion of the superior oblique tendon is searched for *carefully*. At this point, a minimum of manipulation should be carried out; instead, careful blotting with a cotton-tip applicator and slight manipulations of the globe will reveal the insertional fibers of the superior oblique tendon fusing with sclera at approximately right angles to the lateral border of the superior oblique tendon.

B A small muscle hook is then used to engage the superior oblique tendon and bring it temporally. At this point, scissors can be used to dissect the superior oblique tendon free from the intermuscular membrane, fibers, and inferior muscle capsule beneath the superior rectus muscle. Because the superior oblique tendon is fanned out at this insertion, some fibers may be missed at the insertion, but careful dissection beneath the superior rectus will allow complete inclusion of the superior oblique tendon beneath the superior rectus muscle.

C The superior oblique tendon can be brought temporally so that the doubled-over tendon is exposed to a point up to 20 to 24 mm from the insertion. The tenotomy may now be carried out.

D The principle of obtaining more effect from tenotomies closer to the trochlea and less effect from tenectomies farther from the trochlea can be adhered to using the superior oblique exposure from the temporal approach. Since up to 20+ mm of superior oblique tendon can be exposed temporal to the superior rectus, measuring or estimating the distance from the insertion to the point of tenectomy gives actually a more reliable placement of the tenotomy. Since the superior oblique tendon will not stretch, the surgeon should be able to perform a reproducible tenotomy using this technique.

110

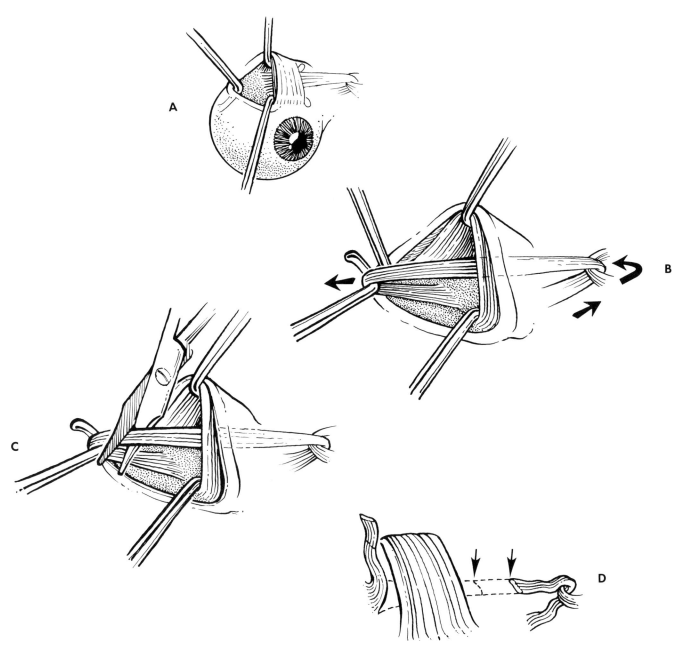

PLATE 7-8

RECESSION OF THE SUPERIOR OBLIQUE

PLATE 7-9

A The superior oblique tendon is located and engaged at its insertion temporal to the lateral border of of the superior rectus.

B A double arm 5-0 Merseline suture is placed through the superior oblique tendon 4.0 mm from its insertion, and a surgeon's knot is tied. The tendon is then transected between the suture and the tendon's insertion.

C The tendon is allowed to retract beneath the superior rectus for a distance of 8 to 20 mm and the suture is tied at the tendon insertion.

Because the superior oblique tendon is a thin structure and is made up of separate, continuous fiber, attempts at marginal tenotomy or tendon splitting–lengthening procedures have been unsuccessful in our hands. In vitro attempts at marginal tenotomy have in our experience produced either no lengthening whatever or transection of the tendon.

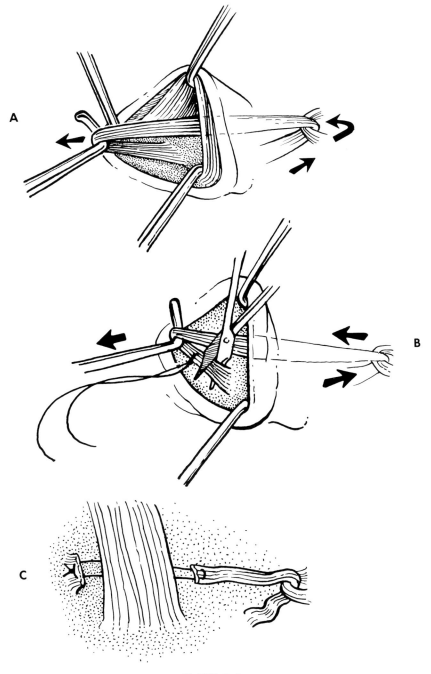

PLATE 7-9

113

SAGITTALIZATION OF THE SUPERIOR OBLIQUE

Sagittalization of the insertion of the superior oblique tendon has been advocated for treatment of the torsional aspect of superior oblique palsy.

PLATE 7-10

A The superior oblique tendon normally inserts in the posterior-temporal quadrant of the globe when viewed from above where it functions as a depressor, abductor, and intorter. By shifting the anterior half of the tendon 5 to 8 mm anteriorly, the intorting action of the superior oblique is enhanced without affecting appreciably the other superior oblique functions.

B The superior oblique tendon is exposed at its insertion, and a Steven's hook splits the insertion.

C The superior rectus is retracted medially, the superior oblique tendon is split, a 5-0 absorbable suture is tied to the superior oblique tendon close to its insertion, and the anterior half of the superior oblique tendon is detached from the globe.

D The anterior half of the superior oblique tendon is sutured to sclera 5 to 8 mm anteriorly, just adjacent to the temporal aspect of the superior rectus.

The anterior superior oblique fibers are probably more effective intorters, and the posterior superior oblique fibers are more effective depressors. A sagittalization effect can be obtained, at least theoretically, by performing a disinsertion of the posterior one half or three fourths of the superior oblique tendon's insertion.

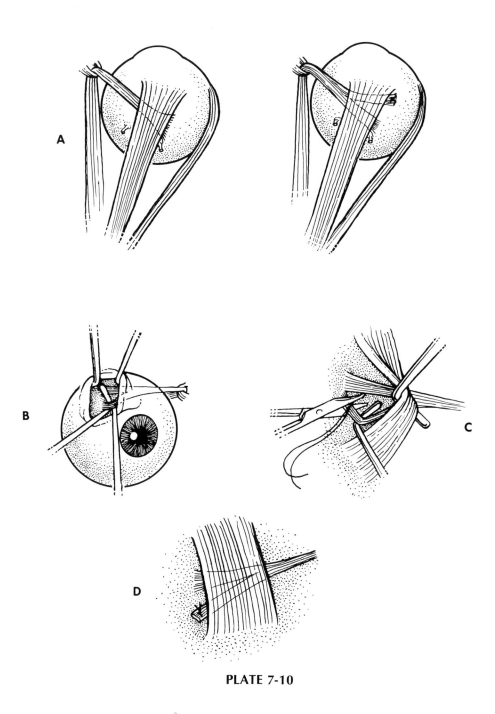

PLATE 7-10

115

Tendon sheath stripping for treatment of Brown's superior oblique tendon sheath syndrome

Brown's superior oblique tendon sheath syndrome is characterized by inability of the eye to elevate normally in the adducted position. It may occur in one eye or both. This syndrome is also associated with widening of the palpebral fissure on attempted elevation. The diagnosis is confirmed by demonstration of limitation of forced elevation, especially in adduction. Brown's syndrome may be congenital or acquired and results from a variety of causes, but the net result is an inability of the superior oblique tendon to pass freely through the trochlea, a function that is necessary to allow the eye to elevate in adduction. Unless the superior oblique tendon can pass freely through the trochlea, the distance between the trochlea and the insertion cannot increase and the eye cannot be elevated in adduction.

The surgical treatment of the superior oblique tendon sheath syndrome is one of the least successful of the extraocular muscle procedures. This is so because surgical attempts designed to reduce the mechanical restriction impeding the normal passage of the superior oblique tendon through the trochlea are often nullified by postoperative adhesion formation. In rare instances, the adhesions that limit elevation in adduction may be associated with structures other than the superior oblique. Girard in such a case has relieved a "Brown's" syndrome by releasing restrictions associated with the inferior oblique, and I have relieved a "Brown's" syndrome by lysing a fibrous band along the inferior border of the lateral rectus.

PLATE 7-11

A The procedure for "sheath" stripping begins by exposing the superior oblique tendon between the trochlea and the medial border of the superior rectus in a manner identical to that done prior to superior oblique tenectomy. The superior oblique tendon and its "sheath,"* from the trochlea to the medial border of the superior rectus, are then examined for abnormal restrictive adhesions.

B Careful dissection is carried out, removing the sheath of the superior oblique tendon from the nasal border of the superior rectus to a point as close to the trochlea as possible. Attempts at elevation of the globe in adduction should be repeated throughout the procedure. Free elevation in adduction indicates successful removal of mechanical restrictions. The superior oblique tendon itself may be cut if restriction to elevation in adduction persists after all associated fascial restrictions have been freed.

C Adhesions forming postoperatively can fix the eye in a position similar to or even worse than was present preoperatively. To avoid this, a traction suture is placed, fixing the eye in an elevated and adducted position. A 4-0 black silk suture is inserted into the episclera in the inferior nasal quadrant. The suture is then brought out through the upper lid and fixed to the brow superiorly and nasally. This suture is tied over a rubber peg and left in place from 5 to 7 days.

---

*Actually the superior oblique has no true sheath. The fascial structures that surround the superior have been called the sheath of the superior oblique erroneously.

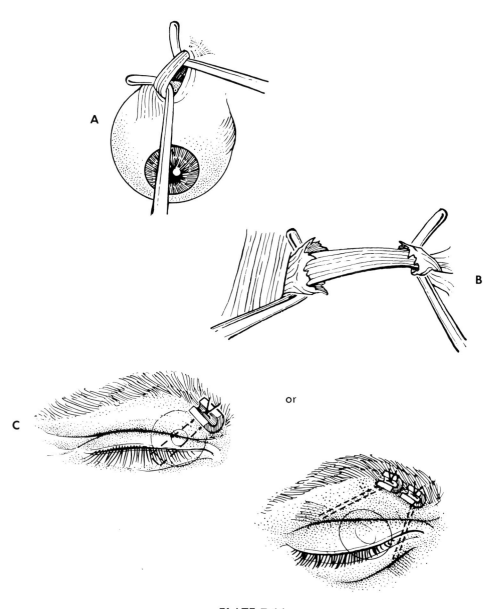

A

B

C

or

PLATE 7-11

117

STRENGTHENING THE SUPERIOR OBLIQUE
Superior oblique tuck at the insertion

The most effective and safest technique for strengthening the superior oblique is a tuck of the tendon at its insertion. This procedure maintains the normal action of the superior oblique muscle and reduces the incidence, severity, and persistence of postoperative Brown's syndrome.

PLATE 7-12

A The incision for exposure of the superior oblique tendon at its insertion is begun at the lateral border of the superior rectus insertion and extends temporally for 6 mm parallel with the limbus. The initial incision is carried through conjunctiva, anterior Tenon's capsule, and intermuscular membrane.

B A muscle hook is inserted behind the insertion of the superior rectus muscle and a second hook retracts the posterior border of the incision at the lateral border of the superior rectus muscle. This maneuver exposes the insertional fibers of the superior oblique tendon.

C A Steven's muscle hook is inserted behind the insertion of the superior oblique tendon, and the tendon is brought out from beneath the superior rectus.

D The Steven's hook is replaced with the hook portion of a Bishop tendon tucker.

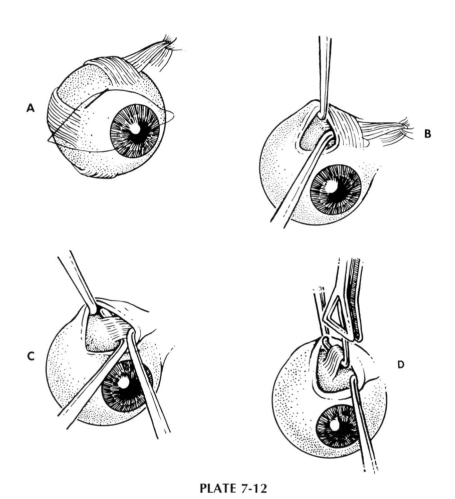

PLATE 7-12

STRENGTHENING THE SUPERIOR OBLIQUE— cont'd
Superior oblique tuck at the insertion—cont'd

PLATE 7-13

A The knurled nut at the head of the tendon tucker is screwed down until the slack has been taken out of the superior oblique tendon. It is impossible to give a number in millimeters for the correct amount of superior oblique tucking in a given case. However, it is safe to say that more errors are committed by doing too small than too large a tuck. I have done tucks ranging from 12 to 22 mm. In general, the more vertical deviation to be treated and the more laxity of the superior oblique tendon, the greater the tuck required. When a sufficient amount of superior oblique tendon has been brought into the tucker so that the slack has been taken out of the tendon, nonabsorbable sutures (my choice is 5-0 Merseline) are then used to anchor the tuck at each border of the superior oblique tendon.

B When each border of the tendon has been secured, the tucker is removed and the tuck remains intact. A third suture is placed at the apex of the tucked tendon, and this tip is attached to sclera in line with the normal pull of the superior oblique tendon. The needle should be placed into very superficial scleral fibers because sclera can be very thin in this area.

C The conjunctiva is closed with several interrupted sutures.

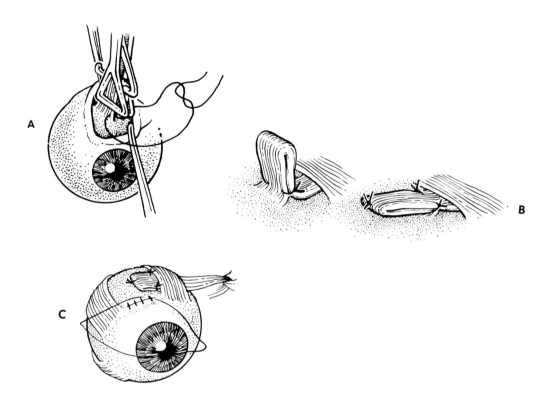

PLATE 7-13

CHAPTER EIGHT

Marginal myotomy: technique and indications

MARGINAL MYOTOMY: HISTORICAL REVIEW

Before the advent of uniform, strong, fine-gauge sutures with sharp swaged-on needles, myotomy was a popular technique for weakening an extraocular muscle. This technique has now been superseded by measured recession, which is the method of choice for weakening the rectus muscles in all but a few specific instances.

PLATE 8-1

Six of the many methods that have been advocated for doing a marginal myotomy are:

1 Central myotomy
2 O'Connor "triple cut" myotomy
3 Incomplete marginal myotomy
4 Overlapping marginal myotomy
5 Multiple incomplete marginal myotomies
6 L shaped overlapping double marginal myotomy

Theoretically types 1, 3, and 5 would not lengthen the muscle, because fibers connecting the origin and insertion of the muscle remain undisturbed. Types 2, 4, and 6 should theoretically lengthen the muscle, but the exact amount of lengthening produced by each technique is impossible to determine from simply observing the artist's drawing.

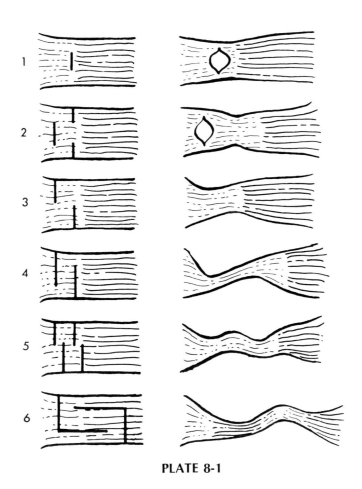

PLATE 8-1

125

QUANTIFYING THE MARGINAL MYOTOMY

The amount of muscle-tendon lengthening produced by a given myotomy was determined in vitro using rabbit eyes enucleated so that 10 to 20 mm of the medial and lateral rectus remained still attached at their insertion.

PLATE 8-2

A The globe muscle preparation was mounted on a specially prepared stand with the muscle held under slight tension parallel to a reference scale. A camera was used to photograph the muscle before and after several different types of tenotomy were performed.

B A double 80% overlapping marginal myotomy produced significant lengthening with shift of the insertion in the direction opposite the point of origin of the proximal (to the insertion) myotomy.

C Incomplete, nonoverlapping, multiple marginal myotomies produced essentially no lengthening.

D A central 80% tenotomy produced essentially no lengthening.

E Two incomplete marginal myotomies combined with an 80% central tenotomy produced moderate lengthening with a symmetrical insertion.

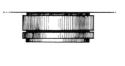

A

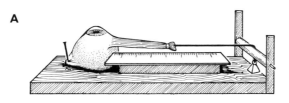

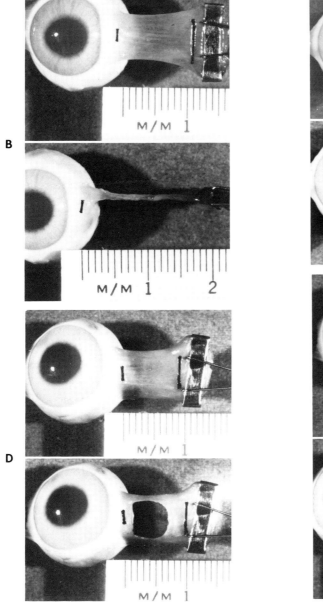

B

D

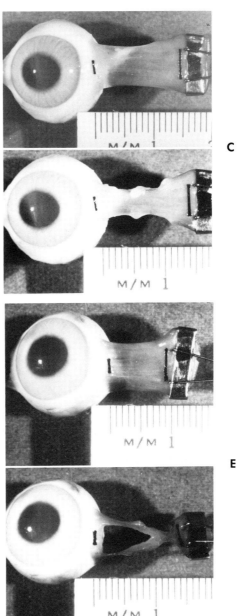

C

E

PLATE 8-2

127

MARGINAL MYOTOMY

Clinically, the most useful of the myotomies discussed here is the overlapping double 80% marginal myotomy.

PLATE 8-4

A The muscle is exposed in the usual manner and two hemostats are each placed 80% of the way across the muscle (or tendon) from opposite borders. The hemostats are placed 3.0 to 4.0 mm apart.

B The posterior hemostat is removed and scissors are used to cut across the muscle in the previously crushed area. By cutting the muscle in the crushed area, bleeding is kept to a minimum.

C The hemostat nearer the insertion is removed and the muscle is cut along the crushed area using small snips with the scissors.

D Noticeable lengthening of the muscle will occur. Any bleeding is controlled with pressure.

The intermuscular membrane at the borders of the muscle should be dissected only far enough to allow placement of the posterior hemostat.

If a *hyperdeviation* is present in an eye treated with such a myotomy of a horizontal rectus, the proximal myotomy should begin above, to shift the insertion downward and make the horizontal rectus more effective as a depressor. If a *hypodeviation* is present, the proximal myotomy should begin below, making the horizontal rectus relatively more effective as an elevator.

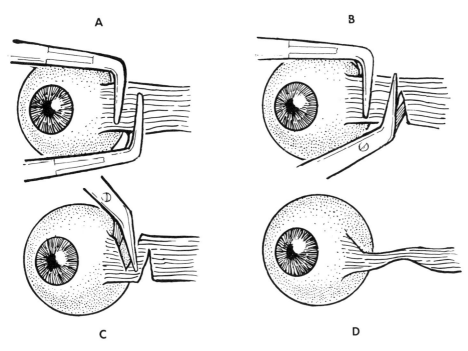

A

B

C

D

PLATE 8-4

131

INDICATIONS FOR A MARGINAL MYOTOMY

There are four indications for doing a marginal myotomy:

1. To further weaken a previously operated rectus muscle that has already been recessed to the functional point of tangency with the globe
2. When combined with a recession, to obtain a double weakening effect while retaining a physiologic arc of contact
3. To weaken a rectus muscle that has at or near its insertion an implant, exoplant, or an encircling element used for retinal detachment repair
4. To weaken a rectus muscle in a patient with excessively thin sclera posterior to the insertion

PLATE 8-5

A   Marginal myotomy performed on an already recessed lateral rectus muscle provides muscle lengthening without sacrificing arc of contact.

B   Left hypotropia has occurred after placement of an exoplant and encircling band near the inferior rectus insertion of the left eye. This has been treated with a double 80% marginal myotomy of the left inferior rectus.

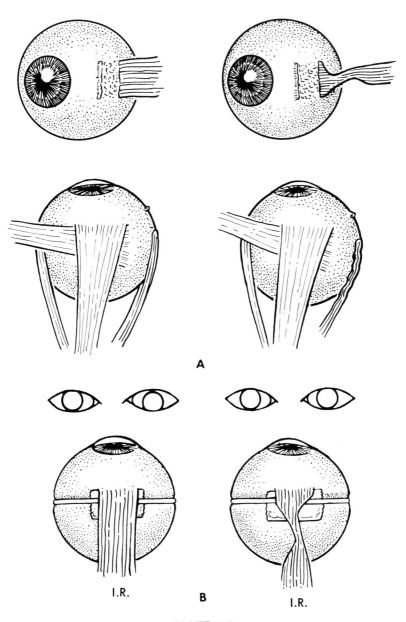

A

B

I.R.   I.R.

PLATE 8-5

CHAPTER NINE

The Faden operation (posterior fixation suture)

The Faden operation was described by Cüppers in Germany and was introduced in the United States by Mulendyck in 1975. A more descriptive term for the Faden operation is *posterior fixation suture* (Faden in German simply means suture). The principle of the posterior fixation suture is to shift the effective insertion of a rectus muscle posteriorly. This theoretically reduces the effectiveness of a muscle so treated in its field of action while there is no effect at all in the primary position or in movement out of the muscle's field of action. Such a mechanical partial crippling of a muscle could be expected to have virtually no effect on the initiation of a movement, but it would have increasing weakening effect the more the eye attempts to move in the field of action of the posteriorly fixated muscle.

The main use for the Faden operation in Europe is in treating the nystagmus blockage (compensation) syndrome, a type of esotropia characterized by (1) variable angle esotropia in childhood, (2) pseudoparalysis of both lateral rectus muscles with nystagmus on attempted abduction, and (3) preference for fixation in adduction while the head turns in the opposite direction, with or without occlusion of the opposite eye, or for fixation with asymmetrical convergence while the head remains straight. In such cases the medial rectus is recessed to treat the static angle and the posterior fixation suture treats the blocking or innervational angle. A posterior fixation suture may also be used in the superior rectus to treat dissociated vertical deviation. Other indications for a posterior fixation suture are chaotic nystagmus and deviations that increase as the eye moves away from the primary position or that are caused only by a secondary deviation.

135

THE FADEN OPERATION (POSTERIOR FIXATION SUTURE)—cont'd

PLATE 9-1

A The posterior fixation suture is placed in sclera and through the muscle, fixing the muscle to sclera at a point behind the equator.

B The point of insertion is shifted posteriorly, thereby reducing the effect of the muscle in its field of action.

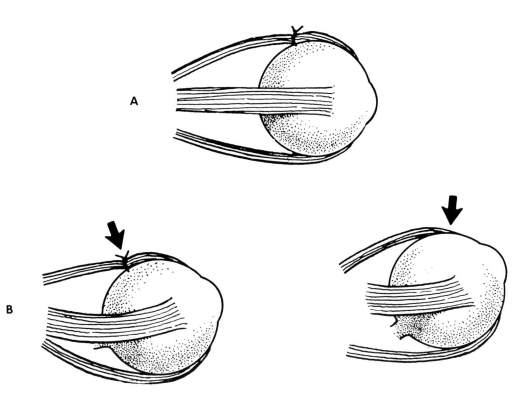

A

B

PLATE 9-1

THE FADEN OPERATION (POSTERIOR FIXATION SUTURE)—cont'd

To be effective, the rectus muscle should be secured to sclera at a point *behind* the equator. This means that the suture is placed approximately 12 mm posterior to the muscle's insertion. This is not an easy suture placement. Vigorous traction must be used to rotate the globe. A thin, ribbon type retractor is useful in retracting the undersurface of the muscle away from sclera. I have performed a Faden operation on the superior, medial, and lateral rectus muscles. The inferior rectus muscle is, in my opinion, the least likely to require a posterior fixation suture and also the most difficult one on which to perform this surgery because of the position of the inferior vortex veins, Lockwood's ligament, and the inferior oblique muscle.

PLATE 9-2

A Posterior fixation suture placement is shown for the superior rectus muscle. The superior oblique muscle is not shown, but if suture placement is carried out properly, sutures are placed at the posterior aspect of the superior oblique insertion. Two double arm 5-0 or 6-0 nonabsorbable sutures may be used to secure the belly of the muscle to sclera, or a single double arm suture may be used.

B The posterior fixation sutures (or suture) are tied securely.

C The muscle is then reattached to its original insertion, or it may be recessed by an appropriate amount, usually between 2.5 and 5 mm.

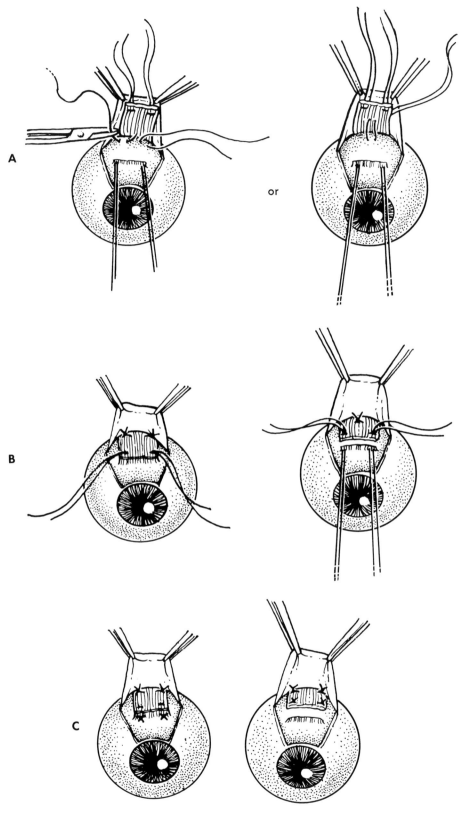

A

B

or

C

PLATE 9-2

THE FADEN OPERATION (POSTERIOR FIXATION SUTURE)—cont'd

The surgeon may wish to place a posterior fixation suture without detaching the muscle.

PLATE 9-3

A After obtaining adequate exposure, the muscle belly is retracted and a suture is placed into superficial sclera approximately 12 mm posterior to the muscle's insertion and is then brought out through the muscle belly.

B Either one or two nonabsorbable 5-0 or 6-0 sutures are tied over the belly of the muscle.

Both the indications for and the results of the Faden or posterior fixation suture are not entirely clear at this time. A posterior fixation suture combined with a 3-mm recession of the superior rectus has been effective in the short term for reducing the manifest part of dissociated vertical deviation. The Europeans have used this procedure extensively for the nystagmus compensation syndrome. I have been able to treat patients with this syndrome effectively and satisfactorily with a large bimedial rectus recession combined with a conjunctival recession.

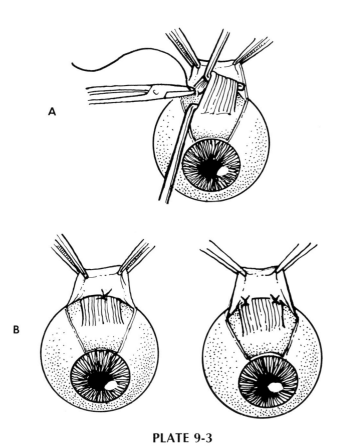

A

B

PLATE 9-3

141

CHAPTER TEN

Diagnostic and surgical techniques for strabismus with restrictions

STRABISMUS WITH RESTRICTED MOTILITY

Excesses or deficiencies of ocular movements can occur as a result of long-standing strabismus as well as of more dramatic and obvious acute palsies or congenital restrictions such as Brown's or Duane's syndrome. Accurate analysis of the sometimes subtle abnormalities in the extent of ocular movement caused by acute or longstanding strabismus is an essential step toward planning the correct surgical procedure. For example, in an esotropic patient with excess adduction in the usually deviated eye and normal ductions otherwise, emphasis should be placed on the medial rectus recession of the deviated eye. Likewise, in a chronically exodeviated eye with excess abduction, emphasis should be placed on recession of the overacting lateral rectus. Deficiencies of ductions are likewise treated by placing emphasis on the resection of the underacting muscle. Manipulation of the amount of recession or resection comprises the "symmetrizing" effect of the recession-resection procedure. Such differences in the amount of surgery between the two eyes can also be employed in so-called symmetrical surgery. In addition to surgery on the muscles themselves, effective use of conjunctival recession, traction sutures, and adjustable sutures can greatly improve the results of surgery in what otherwise would be extremely difficult cases to manage.

STRABISMUS WITH RESTRICTED MOTILITY—cont'd

Congenital or acquired incomitant strabismus with limitations in motility caused by muscle palsies, mechanical restrictions, or a combination of the two are usually easy to recognize. However, proper diagnosis in such cases is absolutely essential before an effective plan for corrective surgery can be determined. Nowhere in strabismus treatment is proper diagnosis more essential to proper execution of surgical skills. The differential diagnosis of strabismus with restricted motility requires analysis of saccadic movements, forced (passive) ductions, and muscle force generation in addition to the usually performed prism and cover tests. The example shown serves as a model for any type of strabismus with restricted motility in one or both eyes and in one or more fields of gaze.

PLATE 10-1

A The patient has a right esotropia in the primary position.

B In levoversion the eyes are grossly parallel, with normal adduction of the right eye and normal abduction of the left eye. No muscle weakness or mechanical restriction is present in this direction of gaze.

C In dextroversion the right esotropia increases markedly. Abduction of the right eye is restricted significantly while adduction of the left eye is normal. The decreased abduction in the right eye could result from a paretic right lateral rectus, a mechanical restriction associated with various muscular or fascial structures in the right eye, or a combination of the two.

144

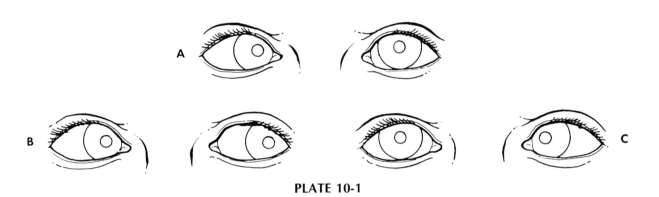

PLATE 10-1

SACCADIC ANALYSIS

PLATE 10-2

A Saccadic velocity analysis begins with the patient fixing on an object in the field opposite that of the suspected paretic muscle. The patient has a right esotropia as shown in Plate 10-1, *A*.

B The patient is asked to switch fixation to an object in the field of action of the suspected paretic muscle. In the case used for illustration the patient is asked to switch fixation from extreme levoversion to extreme dextroversion. During the patient's switch of fixation the examiner observes the speed of the movement in the eye with limited motility, in this case the right eye. If this eye moves at a normal saccadic speed (200° to 400° per second) as does the normal eye, the apparently underacting muscle (the right lateral rectus) is probably contracting in a normal or nearly normal way. The limited motility is probably caused by mechanical restriction associated with this muscle's antagonist or other facial structures around the globe.

C If on the other hand the eye moves to its final position in attempted dextroversion with a slow, floating movement (± 30° per second), there is good evidence that the right lateral rectus is paretic. In this case, little can be determined regarding the presence or absence of associated mechanical restriction.

Saccadic velocity analysis may be done with the aid of an electro-oculograph that provides printed readout.

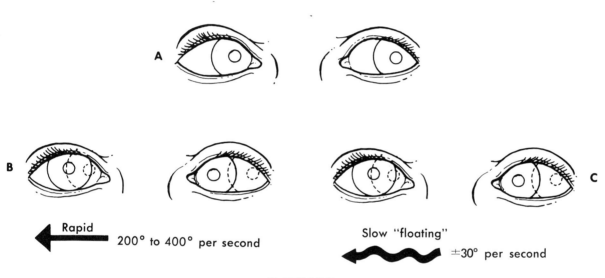

A

B

Rapid
200° to 400° per second

Slow "floating"
±30° per second

C

PLATE 10-2

FORCED (PASSIVE) DUCTIONS

Forced or passive ductions should be carried out on all patients undergoing strabismus surgery. The test is performed in both eyes, in all directions. In most cases forced or passive ductions are done in the operating room just prior to the actual surgery. However, in cooperative patients with restricted motility about whom the surgeon wants as much information as possible before going to the operating room, forced ductions should be carried out in the office using topical anesthesia. Several drops of proparacaine hydrochloride are sufficient to anesthetize the cornea and conjunctiva. A cotton-tip applicator that has been saturated with cocaine hydrochloride 5% is then held against the conjunctiva at the point where the forced duction forceps are to be applied. Fine-toothed forceps are used to grasp the conjunctiva and episclera, and the patient is asked to look *toward* the field of action of the restricted motility. The examiner then gently attempts to assist the eye into the full extent of the attempted duction.

PLATE 10-3

A In the example cited (a patient with a right esotropia and limited abduction of the right eye) the patient is asked to look as far to his right as he can.

B The conjunctiva and episclera of the right eye are grasped with fine-toothed forceps at the nasal limbus (3 o'clock position). The examiner attempts to abduct the right eye gently but forcibly following the normal arc of rotation of the eye around its central vertical axis. If the eye cannot be abducted fully, a mechanical restriction is present and the limitation of abduction results from mechanical causes with or without associated paresis of the lateral rectus.

C If the eye can be abducted fully and the examiner feels no resistance to forced abduction, no mechanical restriction is present and a right lateral rectus paresis is indicated. This finding is always associated with a "floating saccade."

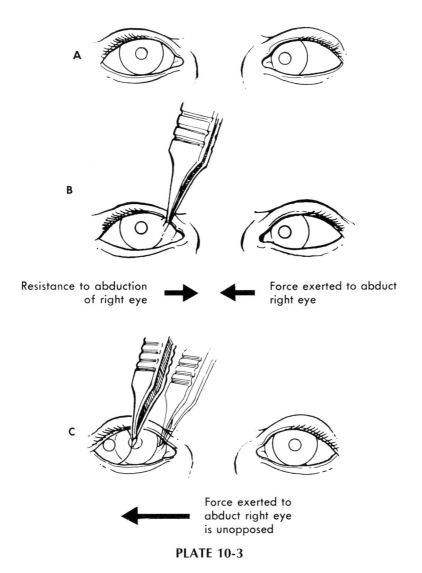

A

B

Resistance to abduction
of right eye

Force exerted to abduct
right eye

C

Force exerted to
abduct right eye
is unopposed

PLATE 10-3

STRABISMUS WITH RESTRICTED MOTILITY

The final step in analyses of strabismus with restricted motility is accomplished with performance of the active, muscle force generation test described by Scott. This test determines, in the presence of restricted eye movements, that amount of force generated by a given extraocular muscle within the range of movement noted on testing of versions and ductions. Active muscle force generation is a tactile test that complements saccadic analysis, a visual test.

PLATE 10-4

A The patient is instructed to look in the direction opposite from the field of action of the muscle to be tested. In the example cited (a right esotropia with limited abduction of the right eye), the patient is asked to look far to his left.

B Several drops of proparacaine hydrochloride (0.5%) are sufficient to anesthetize the cornea and conjunctiva. A cotton-tip applicator that has been saturated with cocaine hydrochloride 5% is held against the conjunctiva at the point where it is to be grasped with the forceps. The anesthetized conjunctiva and episclera of the right eye are grasped with fine-toothed forceps at the nasal limbus (3 o'clock) and the patient is asked to look far to his right while the examiner attempts to stabilize the right eye in extreme adduction. The amount of tug felt by the examiner through his forceps indicates the contracting power of the right lateral rectus. If no appreciable tug is felt, this indicates little if any contraction on the part of the right lateral rectus. This type of response is associated with a floating saccade.

C If the examiner feels a brisk tug on the forceps stabilizing the eye, significant contracting power on the part of the right lateral rectus is indicated. This type of response is associated with a brisk, normal velocity, saccadic movement. The limited movement is therefore caused by a mechanical "leash" or tethering effect usually caused by scar tissue, adhesions, or a spastic, contracted antagonist. More accurate determination of active muscle force generation can be obtained with the use of a strain gauge. Black silk sutures (4-0 or 5-0) are affixed to episclera and are attached to the strain gauge deflector. Isometric contractions should be 60 to 90 gm or more in a normal muscle and are reduced to approximately 10 gm (because of passive tissue forces) in complete paralysis.

The information obtained from saccadic analysis, forced ductions, and the muscle forced generation test helps indicate whether recession-resection and freeing of restrictions is indicated or whether muscle transfer with or without freeing of restrictions is required. When normal contraction with mechanical restriction is present, a recession-resection procedure should be done. When reduced contraction is found, a muscle transfer is indicated.

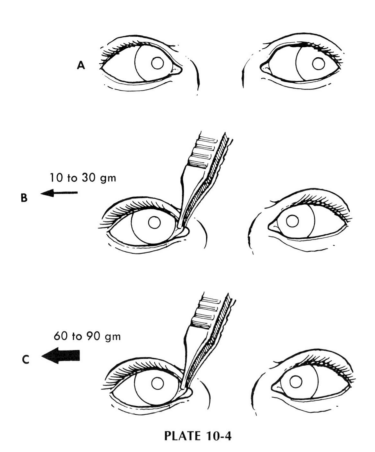

A

10 to 30 gm

B

60 to 90 gm

C

PLATE 10-4

ADJUSTABLE SUTURE TECHNIQUE

The use of adjustable sutures is not new. They were in vogue nearly 50 years ago but fell into disuse only to be rediscovered in recent years. Adjustable sutures find their main use in cases where muscle force is intact but mechanical resistance retards movement of the globe. The two most common clinical situations where the need for adjustable sutures exist are prior unsuccessful surgery and thyroid myopathy. While other situations such as injury cases and resistant strabismus after multiple surgeries that may require the use of an adjustable suture are rarer, any type of strabismus in the presence of adequate muscle force may receive benefit from an adjustable suture. Preoperative postitive force ductions, adequate muscle force generation, rapid saccadic velocity, and the presence of diplopia (and therefore offering hope of a functional cure) are usual preoperative requirements. Because of special anatomical characteristics related to Lockwood's ligament and the inferior vortex veins, adjustable recession of the inferior rectus will be shown. In general, adjustable sutures on any of the rectus muscles are done in a similar fashion.

PLATE 10-5

A After exposure of the inferior rectus is accomplished using the limbal approach, the inferior rectus is engaged with a muscle hook. The intramuscular membrane is dissected 10 mm or more posterior to the insertion with great care being taken to avoid cutting the vortex veins, which are very close to the medial and lateral border of the inferior rectus between 8 and 12 mm posterior to the insertion. Great care must also be exercised in freeing Lockwood's ligament from the outer (closer to the orbit floor) surface of the muscle sheath. This allows a more predictable recession effect with a reduced likelihood of postoperative lid lag.

B After the muscle has been dissected free, a double arm 5-0 Merseline suture is woven through the insertion 1 to 1.5 mm posterior to the insertion.

C A central tie plus a locked loop at each muscle border helps insure suture security in the muscle end.

D Particularly in cases where there is restricted upward movement of the eye, a number 15 Bard Parker blade is used to cut against the muscle hook at the insertion, dissecting the muscle free from its insertion.

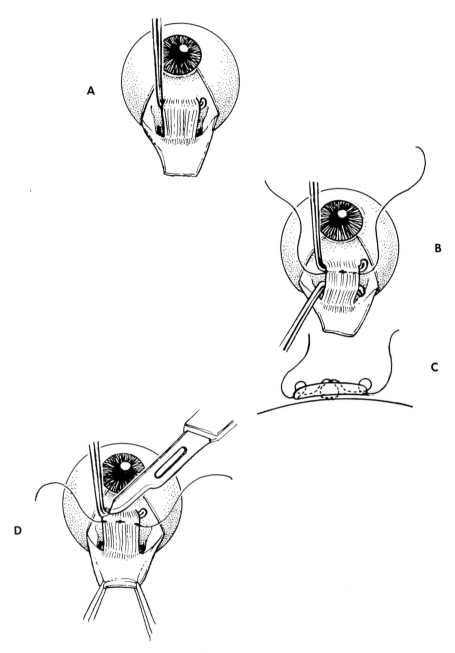

PLATE 10-5

ADJUSTABLE SUTURE TECHNIQUE—cont'd

PLATE 10-6

A After the muscle has been dissected free from the insertion it is allowed to slip backward into the orbit. Each arm of the double arm 5-0 Merseline suture is brought through the muscle stump that has been cut with approximately 1 mm remaining on the globe side. One arm is brought up medially and one arm is brought up laterally.

B The needles are then brought through the fusion of conjunctiva and anterior Tenon's capsule at the edge of this fusion where it had been adjacent to the limbus prior to its dissection. The needles are next brought through a Silastic rod that is 12 mm to 16 mm long, 1.5 mm wide, and 1.0 mm thick. This affects a conjunctiva recession when the suture is tied down and provides a bolster for the suture to be tied over.

C The suture is pulled up and the conjunctiva edge and the bolster are brought down over the muscle's original insertion. The eye is centered in the palpebral opening and, if bilateral surgery is done, is leveled with the other eye. A bow knot is then tied over the bolster.

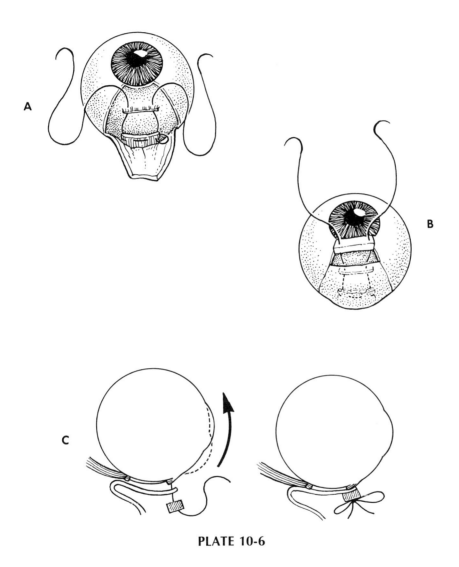

PLATE 10-6

155

ADJUSTABLE SUTURE TECHNIQUE—cont'd

PLATE 10-7

A At the conclusion of the adjustable suture procedure a conjunctival recession has been accomplished with a bow knot tied over the retained Silastic rod.

B The patient is examined on the afternoon following surgery. This is done by close observation, alternate cover testing, and analysis of the subjective responses in the various fields of gaze. If the eyes are not aligned as evidenced by movement on the cover test and diplopia with subjective testing, the bow knot is untied and the muscle is allowed to relax backward in case of a hypodeviation or is brought up forward in case of a hyperdeviation. When the muscle is to be loosened, the patient is asked to look downward after the bow knot has been untied. In cases where bilateral adjustable sutures have been employed, either one or both sutures may be adjusted. Anesthesia is obtained through the use of topical proparacaine hydrochloride. Smooth tying forceps are used to untie and then retie the suture. Adjustment may be done on the morning following surgery and as late as 3 days postoperatively. When the final adjustment on the suture is made, the bow knot is replaced with a surgeons' knot and the excess suture ends are cut. The bolster remains in place.

Ten to 14 days postoperatively the sutures are cut beneath the Silastic bolster and the free ends are allowed to retract beneath the conjunctiva. Adjustable sutures may be employed for any of the rectus muscles, but thyroid myopathy of the inferior rectus is in our experience the most common application for this type of suture. The use of topical anesthesia to preserve muscle funtion for adjustment of the sutures while the patient is on the operating table is unnecessary in our opinion, and in addition we have been unable to find patients who are sufficiently stoic to undergo this type of manipulation.

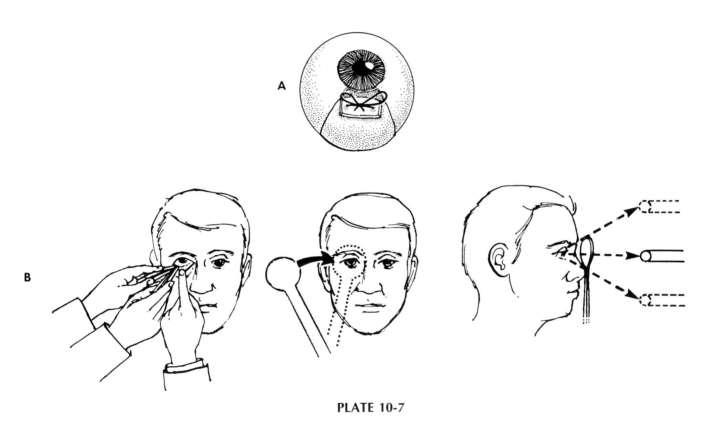

PLATE 10-7

157

SURGICAL TECHNIQUES
Conjunctival recession

PLATE 10-8

A Conjunctival scarring with associated shortening and loss of elasticity of this tissue as well as anterior Tenon's capsule can cause significant restriction in ocular motility. This scarring usually follows surgery in which the transconjunctival approach has been used. Of course, a properly done transconjunctival incision usually does not cause a significant conjunctival scar, but this technique improperly done can cause enough conjunctival restriction so that the effect of properly executed primary or repeat muscle surgery is nullified.

B In order to avoid the restrictive effects of previously scarred or inelastic conjunctiva and Tenon's capsule postoperatively, this fused layer is recessed rather than returned to its preoperative relationship. Sclera is left exposed. The most effective technique for conjunctival recession employs a variation of the limbal incision. The muscle is approached and operated upon in the usual manner. The conjunctival closure is modified by resuturing conjunctiva to sclera just anterior to the insertion of the muscle. This is done using several 5-0 or 6-0 absorbable sutures. The bare sclera will reepithelialize in a few days. This technique frees forced ductions that were previously restricted because of the conjunctiva and causes any scar that may be present to be removed from the center of the palpebral fissure, thereby making it less obvious.

We now routinely employ conjunctival recession in congenital esotropia treated with medial rectus recession. The rationale for this treatment is that long-standing esotropia may cause shortening of the conjunctiva and Tenon's capsule and that if these tissues are returned to their usual position the effectiveness of the medial rectus recession could be decreased or possibly nullified.

158

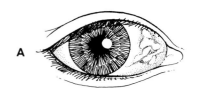 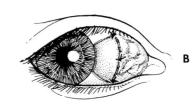

PLATE 10-8

SURGICAL TECHNIQUES—cont'd
Muscle sleeves and implants

PLATE 10-9

A Scarring and adhesion formation between the extraocular muscles, their sheaths, and surrounding structures occur to some extent in all operated muscles. These become more dense in cases where repeated surgery has been done, where suture reaction has been prominent, or when excessive bleeding has occurred during or after the procedure. Since these adhesions have a tendency to recur during repeat surgery, precautions may be taken to avoid their consequences.

B Dunlap has described a Supramid sleeve that may be inserted over the muscle after it has been detached from the globe. This sleeve acts as an artificial sheath that bars formation of unwanted adhesions between the muscle and surrounding structures. Prior to insertion, the sleeve is threaded on a pair of thin forceps or on an alligator forceps.

C The sutures that have been attached to the cut end of the muscle are grasped by the forceps and the muscle is threaded onto the sleeve.

D The sleeve need not be anchored since it cannot advance beyond the new insertion of the muscle. These sleeves may be used with recessions or resections.

E In cases where large segments of the globe are involved in adhesion formation, a curved plate of Supramid may be inserted both above and below the muscle, covering as much as a quadrant.

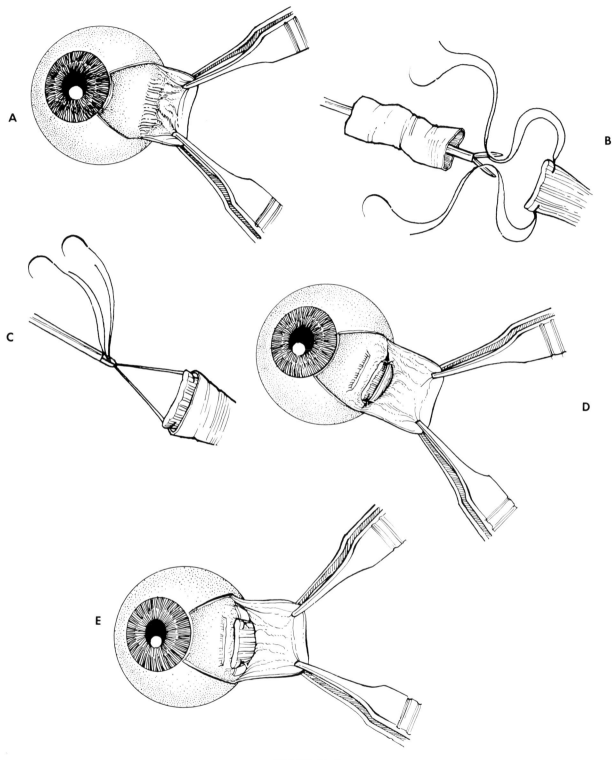

PLATE 10-9

SURGICAL TECHNIQUES—cont'd
Traction sutures

In cases where the surgeon is concerned that postoperative adhesions will cause the globe to remain fixed in an undesirable position, traction suture placement should be employed. The eye should always be placed in a position opposite the undesirable fixation. A chronically esodeviated eye with restricted abduction should be fixed in abduction, a Brown's syndrome should be fixed in adduction and sursumduction, etc.

PLATE 10-10

A This right eye is to be placed in forced abduction. Two scleral bites are taken near the nasal limbus with 4-0 silk sutures.

B The sutures are brought out through the *upper* tarsus and tied over a rubber or silicone peg with the eye in several degrees of abduction. These sutures are removed in 5 to 7 days. Because the eye is abducted, corneal contact by the suture is kept to a minimum. To place the eye in forced adduction, suture placement is reversed.

C To fix the eye in sursumduction two scleral bites are taken at the 6 o'clock limbus and the 4-0 silk sutures are taken out through the *upper* tarsus and tied over a rubber or silicone peg.

D To fix the eye in deorsumduction, the two bites are taken at the 12 o'clock position with 4-0 silk sutures and the sutures are brought out through the *lower* tarsus and tied over a rubber or silicone peg.

E Some surgeons prefer to anchor traction sutures through the tendinous insertion of the rectus muscles. The attachment to the globe is more secure with this technique and the sutures are less likely to be in contact with the cornea. The traction sutures are placed at the insertion of the superior and inferior rectus prior to fixing the eye in abduction or adduction. (Traction sutures are placed at the insertion of the horizontal recti to fix the eye in sursumduction or deorsumduction.) The right eye is fixed in abduction and the sutures are brought out through the *temporal* aspect of the upper lid, fixing the eye in the adducted position.

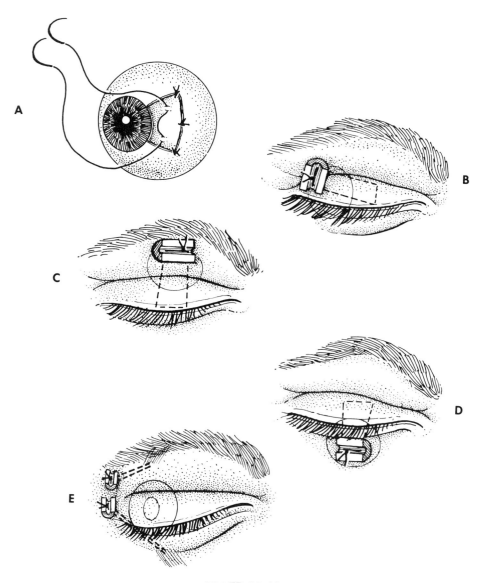

PLATE 10-10

163

CHAPTER ELEVEN

Muscle transposition procedures

When the contractibility of an extraocular muscle is nil, the usual strengthening techniques such as resection, advancement, or tuck do not restore the muscle's potential for ocular rotation. A new, more favorable static position of the globe may be accomplished after a large recession-resection procedure, but movement in the field of action of the paralyzed muscle is not enhanced. Realizing this, Hummelsheim in 1907 devised a procedure to transfer part of the action of the superior and inferior rectus muscles to the field of action of the lateral rectus in cases of sixth nerve palsy.

His procedure has undergone numerous modifications, but the basic principle of most subsequent operations remains the same. The actions of muscles that are normally antagonists are transferred in part to the field of action of the muscle lying between these antagonists: that is, the actions of superior and inferior rectus muscles are in part transferred to the field of action of the lateral rectus in sixth nerve palsy and to the field of action of the medial rectus in partial third nerve palsy affecting the medial rectus. The actions of the horizontal rectus muscles are likewise shifted upward or downward in cases of double elevator or double depressor palsy. The term "muscle transposition" is semantically more accurate than the older term "muscle transplant."

PLATE 11-1

A In Hummelsheim's original "transplant" procedure the lateral halves of the tendons of the superior and inferior rectus muscles are attached to the tendon of the lateral rectus.

B In O'Conner's modification of the Hummelsheim procedure the entire tendon of the superior and inferior rectus muscles is sutured to sclera adjacent to the insertion of the lateral rectus and a cinch is performed on the lateral rectus.

C In a further modification of O'Conner's technique, the nasal half of the superior and inferior rectus tendons are passed beneath the temporal half of the insertions and attached to sclera adjacent to the lateral rectus tendon.

D In Wiener's procedure the paralyzed lateral rectus is transected and the proximal tendon split and joined to the adjacent superior and inferior rectus muscles.

E In Jackson's procedure for third nerve palsy the trochlea is fractured and a shortened superior oblique tendon is sutured to the sclera near the insertion of the medial rectus.

F In Hildreth's procedure the entire tendon of the superior and inferior rectus muscles is joined with nonabsorbable suture.

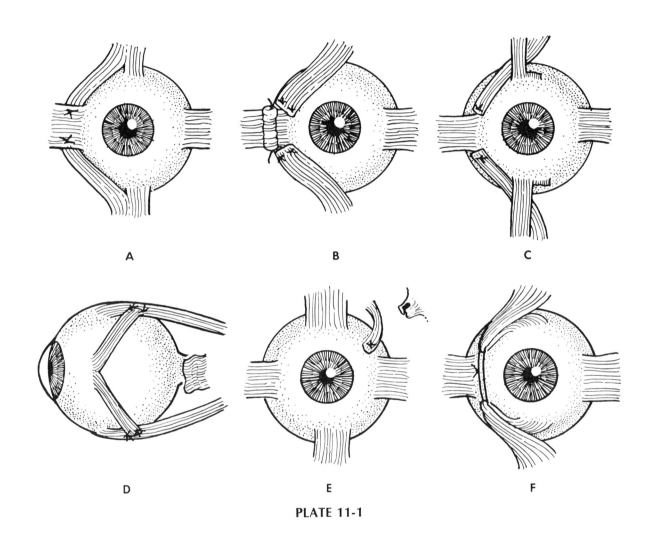

A

B

C

D

E

F

PLATE 11-1

JENSEN PROCEDURE

The Jensen procedure may be employed for paralysis of any of the four rectus muscles. When done for sixth nerve palsy, approximately 30Δ of change in alignment in the primary position may be produced and 20° of rotation in the field of action of the lateral rectus is possible.

PLATE 11-3

A A large limbal incision is made to expose the entire lateral rectus insertion as well as the temporal half of the superior and inferior rectus insertions.

B A Desmarres retractor is used to expose the muscles.

C Each of the exposed muscles is split by bringing a hook through the middle of the insertion. The muscle hook is passed backward toward the muscle's origin for 15 mm.

D A nonabsorbable suture (my choice is 5-0 Merseline) is used to unite the superior half of the lateral rectus and the lateral half of the superior rectus. The knot is tied near the equator. Care must be taken to tie the suture securely but not so tight as to cut through the soft muscle bellies.

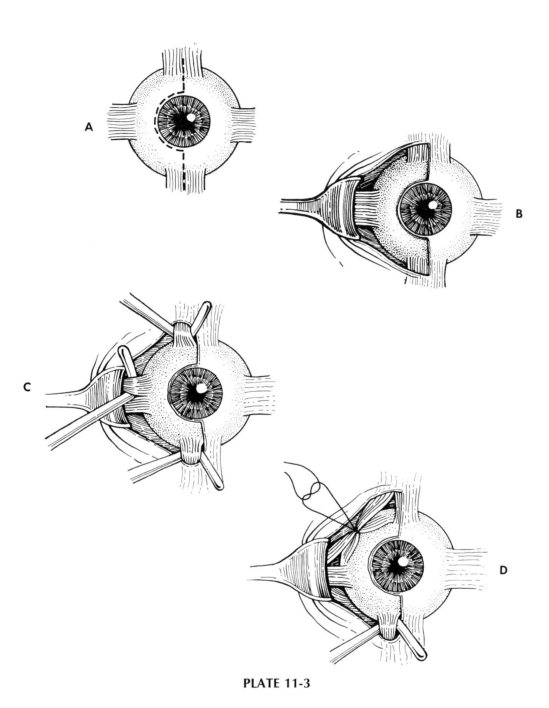

PLATE 11-3

171

JENSEN PROCEDURE—cont'd

PLATE 11-4

A The inferior half of the lateral rectus has been joined to the lateral half of the inferior rectus.

B If the antagonist of the paretic muscle is spastic, causing limited forced ductions in the field of action of the paretic muscle, the spastic muscle should be recessed. The blood supply to the anterior segment remains adequate in spite of the fact that four rectus muscles have been operated upon, because the anterior ciliary arteries in that half of the rectus muscle left undisturbed are still intact. The recessed medial rectus is exposed with a small limbal incision.

C The conjunctiva is closed with several absorbable sutures.

von Noorden has pointed out that anomalous anterior ciliary arteries in the superior and/or inferior rectus may lead to inadvertent ligation of all of the blood supply to the anterior segment supplied through these muscles. The surgeon should inspect and verify the intactness of at least one anterior ciliary artery in each vertical rectus muscle.

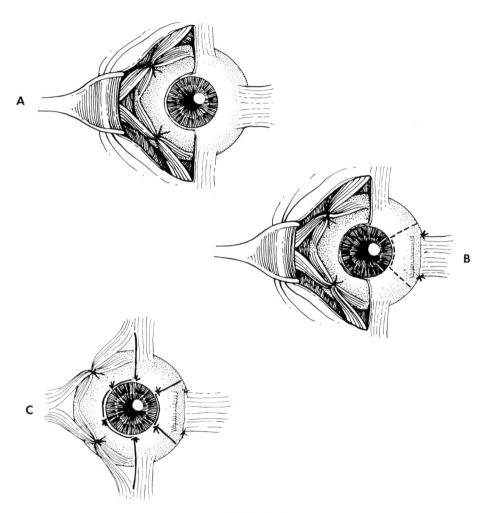

PLATE 11-4

KNAPP PROCEDURE

The Knapp procedure is simple to perform and can produce an average of 38 Δ correction in the primary position and between 25° and 45° of rotation in the field of action of the paralyzed muscle. This technique can also be employed for double depressor palsy, lateral rectus palsy, or partial third nerve palsy involving the medial rectus. In cases where forced ductions are restricted in the field of action of the paralyzed muscle as a result of spastic contraction of the antagonist, this antagonist should be recessed. The repositioning of three of the four rectus muscles with interruption of the anterior ciliary circulation should be done only in young individuals. When recession of the contracted antagonist is required, I ordinarily perform a Jensen muscle transfer procedure.

PLATE 11-5

A   A large limbal peritomy is made, exposing the full extent of the insertion of the muscle to be transferred as well as the insertion of the paralyzed muscle that is the site of the transfer.

B   Sutures are placed just behind the insertion of the two muscles to be transposed in the same way as for a recession. The muscles are detached from the sclera and are resutured at each corner of the insertion of the paralyzed muscle. The antagonist of the paralyzed muscle may be recessed at this point if forced ductions in the field of action of the paralyzed muscle are restricted.

C   The conjunctiva is closed with absorbable sutures.

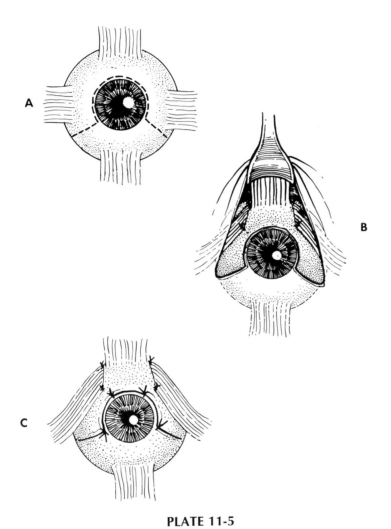

A

B

C

PLATE 11-5

175

SUPERIOR OBLIQUE TENDON TRANSFER

Transfer of the superior oblique can be useful in treatment of complete third nerve palsy. Theoretically the transposed tendon should act more like a tether holding the eye in adduction than a functioning rotator. In spite of this, some adduction results from this procedure and the patient's appearance is improved. Vertical rectus surgery may be indicated at a later procedure.

PLATE 11-6

A A large limbal incision is made from the medial border of the superior rectus to the upper border of the medial rectus.

B The superior oblique tendon is exposed under direct vision and engaged on a muscle hook between the medial border of the superior rectus and the trochlea. This is done in the same manner as with a superior oblique tenectomy.

C A Wheeler canaliculus knife or a fine tip hemostat is passed medially along the superior oblique tendon until the tip is in the trochlea. The knife or hemostat is then used to fracture the trochlea. (The instrument shown is a Wheeler canaliculus knife.)

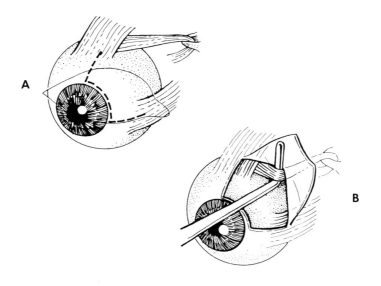

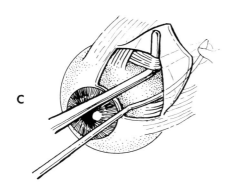

PLATE 11-6

SUPERIOR OBLIQUE TENDON TRANSFER—cont'd

PLATE 11-7

A The superior oblique tendon is pulled free of the trochlea and is transected at the medial border of the superior rectus.

B The eye is placed in a slightly elevated, adducted position and the superior oblique tendon is sutured to the globe just above the superior aspect of the medial rectus insertion using nonabsorbable sutures (my choice is 5-0 Merseline). The superior oblique tendon should be slightly taut, holding the globe in a few degrees of elevation and adduction.

C Excess superior oblique tendon is excised and the conjunctiva is closed with several sutures.

D A large lateral rectus recession should also be done.

In adults the trochlea apparently becomes calcified and is extremely difficult to fracture without also transecting the superior oblique tendon.

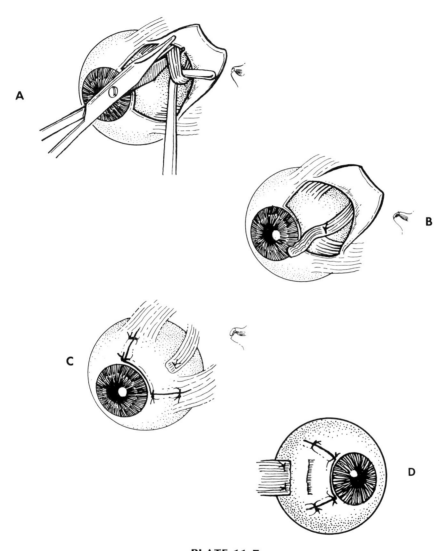

PLATE 11-7

"SUPER MAXIMUM" RECESSION–RESECTION

In certain cases of complete third nerve palsy in adults, particularly those with poor or no vision in one eye, muscle transfer procedures are insufficient. Because of this, I have done a large recession-resection of the horizontal rectus along with a marginal myotomy of the lateral rectus, conjunctival recession laterally, and traction suture placement holding the eye in adduction. Two months later a recession-resection of the vertical recti is done. A rather immobile but well-centered eye has been the result. When cosmetically unacceptable ptosis is present, the intermittent use of crutch glasses may be employed or a ptosis procedure may be done.

PLATE 11-8

A The lateral rectus is recessed 8.0 to 10.0 mm.
B The medial rectus is resected 10.0 to 14.0 mm.
C A double 80% marginal myotomy is done on the recessed lateral rectus.
D A conjunctival recession is done laterally.
E A traction suture holds the eye in the adducted position for 3 to 6 days.

After a 2-month wait, a 5.0-mm recession of the inferior rectus and a 5.0-mm resection of the superior rectus are done.

180

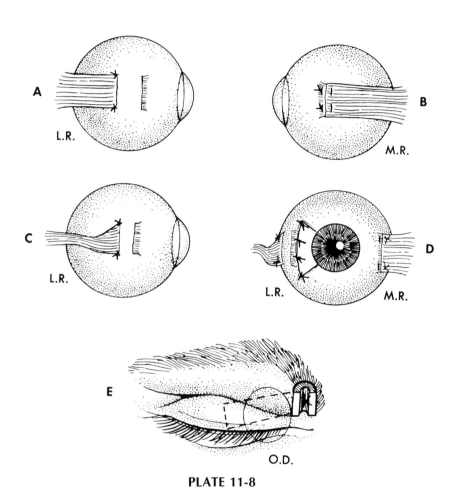

A   L.R.

B   M.R.

C   L.R.

D   L.R.   M.R.

E   O.D.

PLATE 11-8

181

CHAPTER TWELVE

Complications in strabismus surgery

Complications can be eliminated from a surgical practice only by eliminating surgery. This attitude may be fatalistic but it is nontheless accurate. Therefore, surgeons, while realizing that a certain number of complications are inevitable, should always aim at reducing their number and significance. This calls for constant vigilance. The surgeon must be accurate in diagnosis, correct in treatment plan, skillful in execution, and adept at remediation. This chapter lists several complications commonly associated with extraocular muscle surgery (as well as some that are fortunately rare), how to avoid them, and how to treat them when they do occur.

ACUTE, ALLERGIC SUTURE REACTION

Acute, allergic suture reaction occurs with varying severity in approximately 10% and possibly even as high as 20% of patients who undergo strabismus surgery with organic suture material. This reaction presents initially as a dull, red, smooth mass beneath the conjunctiva at the site of the muscle reattachment. The usual postoperative course with uncomplicated primary strabismus surgery in children is for the erythema associated with surgery to be minimal after the first week. In patients who demonstrate a suture reaction, the operated eye shows a significant and fairly sudden increase in redness beginning on the tenth to fourteenth postoperative day. This coincides with the beginning disintegration and absorption of the gut or collagen suture. Clinically apparent acute suture reaction is more frequently associated with resections than recessions because more suture material is used and the sutures are placed nearer the limbus. Acute, allergic suture reaction is not a serious complication. This reaction does not usually alter the outcome of surgery and is self-limiting, subsiding in 2 to 4 weeks if untreated.

PREVENTION

Prevention is virtually impossible in primary cases unless the surgeon routinely uses synthetic, nonantigenic sutures. In cases where suture reaction has occurred with previous surgery, repeat acute, allergic suture reaction can be avoided with the use of synthetic suture, which may be absorbable or nonabsorbable.

Skin testing to aid in finding an organic suture material that will not cause an allergic reaction has been made obsolete by the newer, synthetic absorbable sutures.

TREATMENT

Treatment consists of topically applied steroids. My choice is 0.12% prednisolone twice a day for 7 to 10 days.

CHRONIC SUTURE GRANULOMA

Chronic suture granuloma is fortunately a rare occurrence in strabismus surgery. It appears in less than 0.5% of cases. This reaction is characterized by a solid, red, protruding mass over the site of muscle reattachment. It usually occurs about a week after surgery, beginning before the usual erythema associated with surgery begins to clear. The granuloma is composed of chronic inflammatory cells and fibrous tissue. It may diminish with time but does so slowly and incompletely. Gross undercorrections are frequently associated with this complication.

PREVENTION

Prevention is the same as for acute allergic suture reaction.

TREATMENT

Treatment consists of topically applied steroids; my choice is 0.12% prednisolone twice a day for 2 weeks. If the mass persists it must be surgically excised. Repeat strabismus surgery is often required at this time.

PLATE 12-1

A Acute, allergic suture reaction occurred 12 days after inferior rectus resection.
B After application of 0.12% Prednefrin twice a day for 10 days, the reaction disappeared.
C Chronic suture granuloma persisted 6 months after resection of the lateral rectus.
D The eye looks white and the lateral conjunctiva smooth after excision of the granuloma.

184

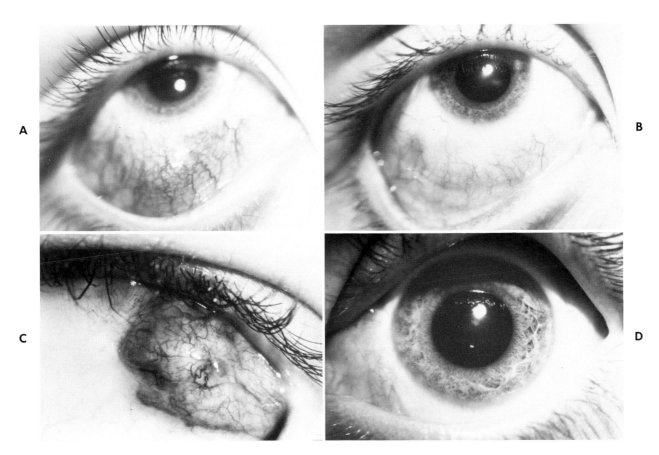

PLATE 12-1

CONJUNCTIVAL CYSTS

Conjunctival cysts may occur when small segments of conjunctival epithelium are buried at the time of conjunctival wound closure. These cysts are usually 2 to 3 mm in diameter and are filled with a clear fluid. They are cosmetically objectionable but do not compromise the results of strabismus surgery.

PREVENTION

Careful closure of conjunctiva at the time of surgery will prevent cysts.

TREATMENT

Evacuation of the cyst may be made with a needle or knife puncture. If this is unsuccessful the cyst must be excised.

PROLAPSE OF TENON'S CAPSULE

Prolapse of Tenon's capsule through the conjunctival incision causes the eye to have an unsightly appearance in the immediate postoperative period. This prolapse is usually caused by incomplete conjunctival closure and is made worse by excess irrigation at the time of surgery. Tenon's capsule under these circumstances tends to imbibe the irrigation solution, thus increasing its bulk.

PREVENTION

Careful wound closure and limited irrigation of the operative site diminishes the possibility of prolapse of Tenon's capsule. If Tenon's capsule is bulky and prolapses in spite of this, any excess may be excised at the time of the initial surgery.

TREATMENT

Prolapsed Tenon's capsule will usually shrink back into the conjunctival wound without active treatment. If the prolapse is excessive and the wound gaping, excess Tenon's capsule should be excised and the conjunctival wound resutured.

PLATE 12-2

A Prolapsed Tenon's capsule persisted 2 weeks postoperatively.
B Tenon's capsule has retracted without treatment 3 months after surgery.

186

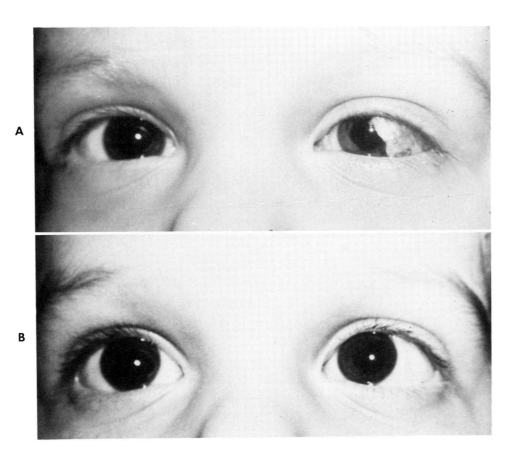

PLATE 12-2

187

SUTURE ABSCESS

A suture abscess occurs as a yellowish elevation over the site of suture placement. It usually occurs within the first week postoperatively. The eye is deeply injected and a purulent drainage may be present.

PREVENTION

Aseptic technique at the time of surgery and routine use of antibiotics postoperatively will prevent suture abscess.

TREATMENT

Treatment includes drainage of the abscess under topical, local, or general anesthesia and appropriate topical antibiotic treatment after culture.

DELLEN

Dellen are small areas of corneal thinning caused by localized drying of the cornea. This corneal thinning does not represent melting away of tissue but rather shrinkage of tissue as a result of local dehydration. The corneal epithelium does not stain but fluorescein will pool in the area, giving the appearance of staining. The localized drying leading to dellen formation is usually caused by elevation of the conjunctiva at the limbus. Dellen were found in 8% of 100 consecutive patients who had extraocular muscle surgery employing the limbus approach. Most were subtle, however, requiring slit lamp examination for diagnosis. Dellen are benign complications that do not affect the outcome of strabismus surgery.

PREVENTION

Smooth closure of the conjunctiva, especially adjacent to the limbus, will prevent delle formation. If decreased tear formation is found preoperatively, patching of the operated eye and/or use of artificial tears should be employed after surgery. Middle-aged women should have a Schirmer test before strabismus surgery.

TREATMENT

Occlusion of the eye for 1 or 2 days will lead to rehydration of the cornea and disappearance of the dellen. Antibiotics may be employed prophylactically while the eye is patched.

PLATE 12-3

A A rather large delle with associated stromal clouding is seen. This clouding is reversible.

B A less obvious delle is adjacent to an area of elevated conjunctiva.

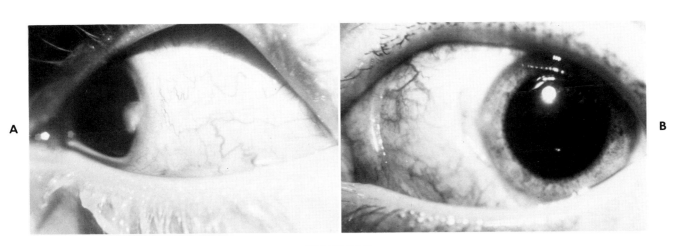

PLATE 12-3

LID FISSURE ANOMALIES

Changes in the vertical dimension of the palpebral opening may occur after recession and resection procedures done on the vertical rectus muscles. Lid displacement following vertical rectus surgery occurs in the same direction as the shift in the insertion of the vertical rectus muscle. Ptosis of the upper lid occurs after excessive resection of the superior rectus. Ptosis of the lower lid occurs after excessive recession of the inferior rectus. Retraction of the upper lid occurs after excessive recession of the superior rectus, and an elevation of the lower lid occurs after excessive resection of the inferior rectus. Excessive resection of either the superior or inferior rectus therefore causes a narrowing of the palpebral fissure, and excessive recession of either the superior rectus or the inferior rectus causes widening of the palpebral fissure. Of the four possibilities, excessive recession of the superior rectus is least likely to cause a lid anomaly.

PREVENTION

Recession and resection of the superior rectus should be limited to 5 mm. Recession and resection of the inferior rectus muscle should not ordinarily exceed 5 mm, but in extreme cases these numbers may be exceeded if careful dissection of the rectus muscle from its surrounding structures is carried out.

TREATMENT

Plastic lid repair is required to treat cosmetically objectionable lid anomalies produced by excessive recessions and resections of the vertical rectus. In the case of a lacerated or slipped muscle, reattachment will improve the lid configuration.

PLATE 12-4

A Ptosis of the left upper lid occurred after excessive resection of the left superior rectus. The surgeon actually intended to resect the left lateral rectus.

B Ptosis of the right lower lid occurred after a 5.0-mm recession of the right inferior rectus without sufficient freeing of the inferior rectus from surrounding structures.

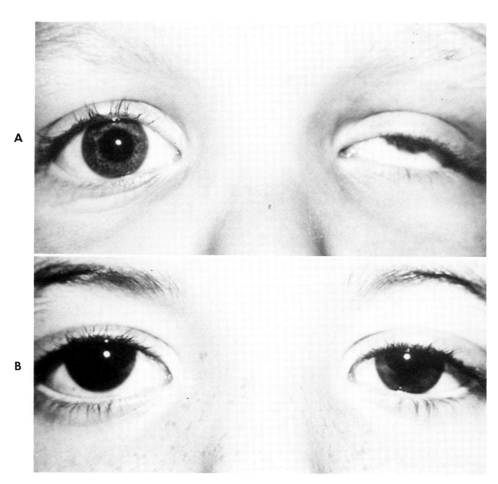

PLATE 12-4

PTOSIS

Ptosis of the medial aspect of the upper lid can occur if the medial part of Whitnall's ligament or the medial horn of the levator muscle of the upper eyelid is torn. This complication is most likely to occur when the superior oblique tendon is hooked medial to the superior rectus using the "blind" technique.

PREVENTION

Exposing and hooking the superior oblique tendon under direct vision will prevent ptosis.

TREATMENT

Repair of the medial horn of the levator muscle is made by the transcutaneous approach.

SCLERAL PERFORATION

Scleral perforation during extraocular muscle surgery probably occurs more often than is realized or reported. Such a perforation may be suspected but not confirmed if the needle used in muscle reattachment or globe fixation seems to pass into and out of the vitreous cavity without incident. On the other hand, the perforation may cause a large defect in the scleral wall with prolapse of uvea and/or vitreous and retinal detachment.

PREVENTION

Sharp spatula needles or very fine (0.008 inch wire diameter) reverse cutting needles should be used for extraocular muscle surgery. These needles should be kept in sight while they are being placed into sclera. In cases of reoperations with adhesions and potentially thin sclera, careful, sharp dissection should be employed. In cases where thin sclera is suspected because of systemic connective tissue anomalies or high myopia, marginal myotomy should be done as a primary weakening procedure to avoid the risk of scleral perforation associated with needle placement for recession. A resection may be carried out safely in such cases by leaving a slightly longer stump at the insertion and using this tissue for muscle reattachment.

TREATMENT

Any time scleral perforation is suspected at the time of surgery, the patient's pupil should be dilated and the fundus over the site of suspected perforation should be examined using an indirect ophthalmoscope. In one case of scleral perforation that I did while attaching the tip of a tucked superior oblique tendon to sclera in a 77-year-old woman, a 0.5 mm dot of hemorrhage was seen. No treatment was given. Over the next 12 months, a 1.0 mm atrophic scar was observed. It has not undergone further change in another year and no other retinal abnormalities have been observed. Some surgeons prefer to treat inadvertent scleral perforations with application of cryotherapy, diathermy, or even a scleral buckle for support.

Simple perforations without prolapse of vitreous or uvea may be left untreated. If uvea or vitreous prolapses or if the defect is large, it should be closed with sutures and a ring of cryothermy or diathermy should be placed around the site of perforation. The extraocular muscle procedure should be suspended at that time.

SLIPPED OR "LOST" MUSCLE

A slipped or lost muscle may occur at the time of surgery or may be noted in the first hours or days after surgery. When this complication occurs during surgery, the muscle can usually be found without much difficulty and the intended surgery carried out. If a recession is being done, irrigating solution flowing freely into the area of the slipped muscle will usually cause the cut end of the tendon to be evident as a whitish structure. The muscle may then be grasped and resutured. Slippage in a resected muscle noted at the time of surgery is more difficult to remedy because the surgeon is dealing with a shortened muscle without a tendinous tip. However, with careful "hand over hand" grasping of tissue in the area, the muscle can usually be found and reattached. A slipped muscle occurring after the patient has left the operating room is an embarrassing and often troublesome complication. It is easily diagnosed because the patient is unable to move the eye in the field of action of the slipped muscle. This condition is associated with either a marked overcorrection in the primary position or a deviation of greater magnitude than appeared preoperatively.

PREVENTION

Slipped muscles are prevented only by exercising proper care in the operating room at the time of surgery. Knots should be tied securely and suture bites into sclera should be made sufficiently deep to ensure proper anchoring of the muscle.

TREATMENT

Treatment of loss of a muscle in the operating room has been discussed. Slippage of a muscle occurring after a patient has left the operating room is an indication for *immediate* return of the patient to the operating room. Careful search for the muscle should be carried out, and if the muscle is found it should be resutured in the way that was intended initially. If a muscle cannot be found, suturing Tenon's capsule to the muscle's insertion can be done but is rarely helpful. An electric muscle stimulator designed by Alan B. Scott may be employed to aid in finding a lost muscle. Electrical stimulation in orbital tissue causes muscle tissue to "twitch," rendering it identifiable in contrast to other nonmuscular but often similar appearing orbital tissue. A muscle transfer procedure may be necessary.

ANTERIOR SEGMENT ISCHEMIA

Corneal clouding, stromal swelling and wrinkling, and heavy flare and cell reaction in the anterior chamber may occur, especially in elderly patients, after extraocular muscle surgery. Detachment of two adjacent rectus muscles may cause segmental iris atrophy. Detachment of three or four rectus muscles or performing a Jensen procedure in an adult or elderly patient may cause severe anterior segment reaction. von Noorden has pointed out the possibility that anterior ciliary arteries if they follow an aberrant course may be inadvertently obliterated

193

in performing the Jensen muscle transfer procedure. In addition to iris atrophy, anterior segment ischemia has resulted in cataract formation. The corneal reaction usually clears, but iris atrophy and cataractous changes usually persist after the acute anterior segment ischemia subsides.

PREVENTION

All four rectus muscles should never be detached in any patient. In adults or elderly patients detachment of adjacent rectus muscles should be done only when deemed absolutely necessary. Complete detachment of three rectus muscles should not be done in an adult patient. When a Jensen procedure is being performed in an adult patient, great care should be taken to ensure that at least one anterior ciliary vessel remains intact in each of the antagonist muscles that has half of the muscle belly shifted.

TREATMENT

Topical steroids such as 1% prednisolone several times a day, systemic steroids between 50 and 100 mg for 10 days, and 1% atropine drops twice a day to dilate the pupil comprise the usual treatment routine.

SUPERIOR RECTUS DENERVATION

Superior rectus denervation may occur if the muscle hook is thrust too deeply into the globe at the time of superior oblique surgery.

PREVENTION

Hooking the superior oblique under direct vision will prevent this.

TREATMENT

Treatment consists of waiting 6 to 9 months for recovery of function, and then either a recession-resection of the vertical rectus muscles or a muscle transfer procedure is done.

PERSISTENT OVERACTION OF THE INFERIOR OBLIQUE

Persistent overaction of the inferior oblique may occur if some of the inferior oblique fibers have been left intact.

PREVENTION

Careful exposure of the posterior aspect of the inferior oblique muscle should be carried out routinely. Any remaining fibers should then be transected. It has been said that the inferior oblique may have two or three heads. However, this possible anatomic variation is of no significance if myectomy is done in the inferior temporal quadrant.

TREATMENT

The inferior oblique must be explored and reweakened using the surgeon's favorite technique.

194

OPERATION ON THE WRONG EYE

PREVENTION

It should be determined preoperatively which eye is to be operated on, and the patient's records should be brought to the operating room. Very frequently in horizontal rectus surgery it makes very little difference which eye is operated on. In this case, parents should be told that either eye may be operated upon but the final decision will depend upon forced ductions, which are done in the operating room.

TREATMENT

If the wrong eye had a horizontal recession-resection, probably nothing should be done. If vertical surgery has been done on the wrong eye the deviation will be made worse. If the error is discovered in the operating room, the surgery should be reversed and the proper surgery done. If wrong eye surgery is discovered postoperatively, the patient should be treated as a new case and reoperated according to the findings.

OPERATION ON THE WRONG PATIENT

PREVENTION

A surgeon should know his patient. The patient's hospital identification should be checked to make sure the patient matches the records.

TREATMENT

In such a case the patient should be treated as a new patient.

ORBITAL CELLULITIS

Orbital cellulitis is a rare but most unfortunate complication following extraocular muscle surgery. Proptosis, extreme redness, chemosis, and pain with lid swelling characterize this complication, which may occur during the first week to 10 days postoperatively.

PREVENTION

Aseptic technique prevents orbital cellulitis.

TREATMENT

Culture and sensitivity determination should be done and the proper systemic and topical antibiotic treatment carried out. A broad-spectrum antibiotic may be used prior to receiving the specific laboratory results. It is probably best to treat such patients in the hospital with the help of a pediatrician or an internist.

PANOPHTHALMITIS

Panophthalmitis is fortunately an extremely rare occurrence after extraocular muscle surgery.

PREVENTION

Aseptic technique will prevent panophthalmitis.

TREATMENT

Treatment consists of appropriate topical and systemic antibiotic therapy with steroids. If the eye is destroyed, evisceration must be carried out.

BROWN'S SUPERIOR OBLIQUE TENDON SHEATH SYNDROME

Brown's superior oblique tendon sheath syndrome may occur after a superior oblique tuck. If the tuck is done at the insertion, no mechanical reason for a typical Brown's syndrome exists. We have done forced ductions on patients with postoperative "Brown's syndrome" and have found the forced ductions to be free under anesthesia. This leads us to believe that, at least in certain cases, a "Brown's syndrome" after superior oblique tuck results from spasm of the muscle rather than from an inability of the tendon to pass freely through the trochlea.

PREVENTION

The superior oblique tendon is tucked only at the insertion and tucks of excessive amount are avoided; that is, the superior oblique tendon should be tucked only to the point of being snug. My maximum tuck to date has been 22 mm.

TREATMENT

With time, a properly done tuck will in most cases cease to cause a "Brown's syndrome." If after several months the eye does not elevate well in adduction and diplopia is bothersome, the superior oblique tuck done at the insertion should be taken down. If the tuck has been done between the trochlea and the medial rectus, it should be taken down and treated as a primary Brown's syndrome.

SYMBLEPHARON

Symblepharon may occur with improperly placed conjunctival incisions.

PREVENTION

Careful conjunctival incision and closure will prevent symblepharon.

TREATMENT

Conjunctival recession with bare sclera closure should be carried out if ocular motility is restricted or if the conjunctiva is reddened and unsightly.

ORBITAL HEMORRHAGE

Orbital hemorrhage may occur after a vortex vein is cut or when a patient has an unrecognized blood dyscrasia. Cutting a vortex vein causes a large, usually anterior, hematoma that results in unsightly lid swelling and ecchymosis. Blood dyscrasias cause a far more serious, generalized oozing into all orbital tissue. In one operation that I did, which resulted in generalized orbital hemorrhage, 8 mm of proptosis occurred in both eyes along with intraocular pressures elevated to near 50 mm Hg, corneal edema, and easily induced retinal artery pulsations.

196

PREVENTION

Careful dissection, coupled with awareness of the location of the vortex veins, can reduce or eliminate hemorrhages from this cause. Blood dyscrasias should be uncovered preoperatively in the course of securing an adequate history. In any case where a bleeding tendency is suspected, hematologic evaluation should be obtained.

TREATMENT

A severed vortex vein should be controlled with local pressure over the bleeding site. No cautery should be used. The treatment of orbital hemorrhage from blood dyscrasia is centered around the surgeon's attempts to maintain a reasonable intraocular pressure during the acute period. Fortunately, children and young adults can withstand brief periods (up to several hours) of very high intraocular pressure without sustaining damage. If such a hemorrhage occurs, osmotic agents and digital massage along with careful monitoring of the intraocular pressure are indicated. Such hemorrhages occurring after extraocular muscle surgery should not be treated with paracentesis.

PLATE 12-5

A 28-year-old male developed a diffuse orbital hemorrhage during surgery that consisted of a recession of both lateral rectus muscles 7.0 mm and resection of the right medial rectus muscle 8.0 mm. This photo was taken 24 hours after surgery. The intraocular pressure, which had been near 50 mm Hg in each eye, had reduced to approximately 25 mm Hg. Proptosis had diminished from 8 to 2 mm, and the corneas had cleared. The patient underwent a total recovery and obtained an excellent surgical result.

UNDESIRABLE OVERCORRECTIONS AND UNDERCORRECTIONS

Undesirable overcorrections and undercorrections are an inevitable accompaniment of the practice of surgical treatment of strabismus.

PREVENTION

A careful, accurate workup, correct choice of surgery, and proper execution of surgery will reduce a surgeon's undesirable overcorrections and undercorrections. The percentage of cases corrected to within ± 10Δ of the intended postoperative angle will depend on the preceding factors and also on the surgeon's ability to learn from past experience. Since similar types of patients react in similar ways, the surgeon should not make the same "mistake" repeatedly. It should also be emphasized that by overcorrection or undercorrection I mean more or less correction than the surgeon *intended*. This is significant, because some categories of patients should be undercorrected relative to ortho position and others should be overcorrected.

TREATMENT

Overcorrections or undercorrections should be treated according to Cooper's dictum, that is, as though they were new cases, with appropriate medical, optical, orthoptic, or surgical remedies employed. In addition, the surgeon should rely on force and velocity studies in the planning of secondary surgery.

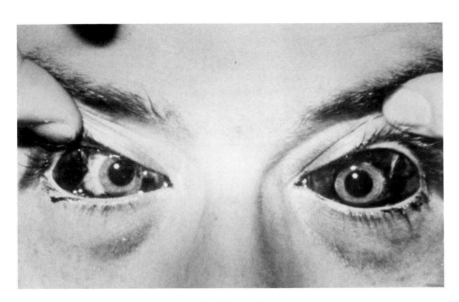

PLATE 12-5

Surgical overcorrections — Board qu.

I. XT treated c̄ Surgery → Consecutive ET of 25△ — Blindspot-Syn.
Postop:- Immediately —
① Patching → alternately each eye patched c̄ bilat. recess
→ operate amblyopic eye patched in R & R.

② Prisms — if no response c̄ patch
— divide equally between two eyes — in bilat. recess
— 20 : 5 △ in R & R.
      amblyopic
      eye
③ Glasses
④ Surgery.

II Undercorrection —
ET → post-op still ET
① Patching if amblyopic +
② Miotic or glasses
③ Prisms ?
④ Surgery if indicated.

III Eccentric fixation —
① Patch preop
② Do surgery for amount of stabismus
③ Patch good eye on table so that pt. wakes up c̄ bad eye straight

IV XT c̄ amblyopia → overcorrected slightly post operative put prisms
for cosmetic appearance & the glasses also act as a protection for good eye

V XT corrected c̄ Bilat. recession → Still XT Post op → yrs ago.
                 Rx → marginal myotomy of lat. rectus c̄
                        resection of M.R.

VI XT Corrected c̄ R & R one eye → Still XT Post op →
                 Rx — R & R on other eye.

VII Secondary XT — following Correction of ET → See page ⑯ in
                                                     Atlas of Strabismus
Do a duction test —
→ if the lat. rectus is resected too much, the eye will not
move i.e. tight lat. rectus will act like a leash → Recession
                                                     or marginal m.
→ if the eye has deficient adduction → Leave   of rectus
unrestricted passive adduction. → Shows that med. rect.
was excessively recessed.   Rx — med. rectus should be advanced
                                  to the original insertion & Resected

Advancement & resection is a strong procedure.
eg:- 25 XT — do 5 mm advance + 2 mm resect. If more than 5 mm
advancement necessary do not resect. There are no definite
numbers for this Surgery.

⑳⓪.

CHAPTER THIRTEEN

A logical scheme for the planning of strabismus surgery

DESIGN OF THE SURGICAL PROCEDURE

At the outset it was said that no attempt would be made to present a set of surgical recipes resulting in a predetermined amount of straightening. This intent remains. However, there are certain principles that have proved helpful to me in the surgical management of strabismus. These will be presented in the form of useful guidelines. These guidelines are general rather than dogmatic, but when properly applied to a specific case, they help assure that the chosen surgical procedure will be "custom tailored" to that individual and to his strabismus problem. This plan for surgery must be arrived at in a dynamic fashion. To do this, the three basic components contributing to the ultimate surgical design should be determined accurately, understood thoroughly, and combined logically. When these logical but simple steps are carried out, the answers to the questions: *which muscle?* and *how much surgery?* should be obvious to the surgeon.

The first task that must be accomplished by the ophthalmologist in the quest for successful surgical treatment of strabismus is to record a pertinent history and compile an accurate, complete set of measurements, including an accurate cycloplegic refraction. This latter, often underrated, component of the strabismus evaluation is especially important if any hyperopia is present in a patient with an esodeviation. If any question remains regarding the accuracy of the cycloplegic refraction, it should be repeated until accuracy is assured.

The second prerequisite is that the surgeon be aware of all of the surgical options available to him. He must also know approximately how much change in ocular alignment he can expect ot produce with each procedure in *his own hands.*

The third step in the design of the surgical procedure joins steps 1 and 2 and comprises the "art of strabismus surgery." This aspect of the surgical design deals with how various types of patients and various categories of deviations repond to given amounts of surgery. The *anticipated* response in a given patient, therefore, modifies the results to be expected from a particular procedure. Also, the most desirable end result that could be obtained from surgery, such as slight overcorrection or undercorrection, can be determined after careful analysis has led to a thorough knowledge of the patient. For example, a patient with a large deviation will obtain more correction per millimeter of surgery than a patient who has a smaller deviation; esotropic patients with amblyopia may be overcorrected with the same amount of surgery that would produce an undercorrection

201

in a free alternator; patients with fusion potential should be slightly overcorrected, patients without fusion potential should usually be undercorrected, and so on. This extra bit of insight as to how a particular type of patient will respond to a given amount of surgery helps the surgeon to combine each individual patient's needs and the type and amount of surgery required. In this way, the maximum benefit from surgery is provided for each patient.

It should be understood that all appropriate nonsurgical techniques that would eliminate the need for surgery or enhance the results obtained from surgery should be carried out. This includes such measures as the correction of hyperopia in esotropic patients who are suspected of having an accommodative element to their esotropia and use of prisms, anticholinesterase drops, and suitable orthoptic exercises. A detailed discussion of nonsurgical treatment of strabismus is beyond the scope of this book.

Step 1: Patient evaluation

The initial workup may be recorded on a preprinted sheet similar to the one illustrated in Plate 13-1. The following questions should be answered and the indicated tests performed and recorded during the process of patient evaluation prior to strabismus surgery.

History:
    Why was the patient brought in
        (why did he come in) for examination?
    What have the parents (what has the patient)
        noted about the eyes?
    Age of onset
    Current age
    Birth weight
    Growth and development
        Present weight
        Sat up when*
        Walked when*

Symptoms:
    Diplopia (do things tilt?)
    Asthenopia
    Other

Occlusion:
    Which eye
    How long
    How well

Orthoptics:
    Type of exercises
    How long
    How well

Family history:
    Strabismus
    Glaucoma
    Diabetes
    Other eye problems

General health:
    Trauma
    Diabetes
    Fatigability†

Habits:
    Head tilt
    Preferred eye
    Variability of deviation

Prior treatment:
    Glasses
        When prescribed
        Prescription
            Bifocals
            Prisms

Surgery:
    When
    What was done
    By whom

*Of interest primarily in infants and young children.
†Especially important in suspected myasthenia.

202

OCULAR MOTILITY EXAMINATION

AGE ONSET	HX:	AGE NOW	

GLASSES (/ /)   OCCLUSION   ORTHOPTICS   SURGERY

OD
OS
        ADD

VISION	"E" GAME	LINEAR "E"	LETTER CHT.	PIN HOLE	OTHER
OD	/	/	/	/	/
OS	/	/	/	/	/

FIXATION   DUCTIONS   SCREEN COMITANCE

HEAD POSTURE

AMBLYOSCOPE   RANGE   SUPP.

OBJ. =   /   TO   /   SUPERIMP.

SUB. =   /   TO   /   FUSION

STEREO   WORTH   BAG.   A.I.

PRISM COVER TEST

DIST. $\bar{s}$ GL. =

DIST. $\bar{c}$ GL. =

NEAR $\bar{s}$ GL. =

NEAR $\bar{c}$ GL. =

FIXATION

DIAGNOSIS

TREATMENT

_____ M.D.
                        SIGNATURE

RETURN APPT. _____ DATE _____

OCULAR MOTILITY EXAMINATION

PLATE 13-1

203

VISUAL ACUITY TESTING

With an infant or a child too young to cooperate for visual acuity testing, reaction to a light, a nonilluminated (silent) interesting object, social situations, and, if poor vision is suspected, an opticokinetic tape or drum should be observed. Notation is made describing the best acuity observed: for example, "appears to be (not to be) visually alert to _____ (a note made as to the size of the smallest object seen)." Strong preference for one eye associated with objection to occlusion of this eye usually indicates amblyopia or an organic visual defect in the other eye. Cross fixation, on the other hand, rules out amblyopia.

Visual acuity testing with an E chart or a STYCAR chart can usually be accomplished at the earliest with girls at age 3 and boys at age 3½, although exceptions do occur. Linear testing with E's or letters is valid. Testing with isolated E's gives erroneously good vision in the presence of functional amblyopia beause of the absence of the crowding phenomenon. Isolate. E's are used in Indiana University Clinic only for instruction. Vision in older children is determined with the letter chart. In children where testing with the E chart cannot be accomplished, pictured cards designed by Henry Allen, M.D., are used at distances of 10 feet or less. As a screening device for fusion, as well as vision, Reinecke has suggested the use of a random dot stereogram.

When decreased vision occurs in both eyes, vision should be checked binocularly and latent gross or micronystagmus should be looked for. Fogging with plus lenses may be used to block vision in one eye while determining monocular visual acuity in patients with latent nystagmus. Near vision should be checked with E's, isolated letters or sentence reading, depending on age. Visual acuity testing with neutral density filters can differentiate functional from organic amblyopia. Vision in an eye with functional amblyopia remains at or near the same level when neutral filters of increasing density are introduced before it, while vision in an eye with organic amblyopia decreases proportionally with the increased density of the filter. Near point of accommodation is determined in cooperative patients by moving a card with small print closer to the patient until the blur point is reached. The near point of accommodation is recorded in diopters or centimeters.

MOTOR EVALUATION

Fixation. Which eye is preferred for fixation? If neither eye is preferred and the eyes appear grossly straight, fusion may be present or at least apparent. If so, the word "fusion" is recorded. In the presence of strabismus, if one eye is preferred for fixation and the other eye deviated, the notation is: "fixation OD" or "fixation OS." Free alternation or cross fixation may be present and is recorded as such. A patient may prefer one eye but hold fixation briefly with the nonpreferred eye after the cover has been removed from the preferred eye. This is recorded: "prefers OD, will hold but not take up fixation OS." Gross, wandering fixation may be present in the nonpreferred eye and should be recorded as such. Nystagmus, if present, is noted and characterized such as latent or manifest, horizontal, rotary, vertical, pendular, jerk, and the like. Nystagmoid movements differ from nystagmus in that the former are nonrhythmic.

Ductions. Ductions or monocular movements are evaluated in extreme abduction, adduction, sursumduction, and deorsumduction. Ductions are graded 1+ to 4+ overaction or underaction, according to the examiner's own system. Forced ductions, muscle force generation, and saccadic speeds are determined in patients with significant limitation of ductions.

Head posture. Any face turn or head tilt is noted and recorded. This is an especially helpful clue in patients with vertical muscle palsies and with strabismus with limitation of ductions where fusion is present. A bizarre head posture may be assumed to aid in fusion or to increase the amount of diplopia to aid suppression.

Screen comitance. Versions, or binocular eye movements, are evaluated in the extreme cardinal positions. Arrows and hash marks on the record indicate overaction or underaction of the muscles. Arrows outside the figure indicate overaction and hash marks on the lines denote underaction. The lines in the H figures represent the field of action rather than the location of the six extraocular muscles of each eye.

SENSORY EVALUATION

In selected cases, certain sensory tests should be done after the history has been taken but even before visual acuity has been determined. The type of patients in this category are those who fuse in everyday casual situations that are not stressful but who lose their weak hold on fusion after even the slightest dissociation. Patients with any type of intermittent deviation and bifoveal or peripheral fusion should have their stereoacuity determined initially and then should be tested with the Worth four dot test before resuming the more usual flow of the examination. In addition, stereoacuity testing is a good screening device for suspected normal patients. Any patient who accurately sees nine out of nine Titmus vectographic targets is unlikely to have much wrong with his binocular mechanism.

First-degree fusion

The objective angle is the patient's manifest or latent strabismus (deviation), as determined by the examiner using the major amblyoscope. This is essentially the same angle found with alternate prism and cover testing. The subjective angle is the angle at which the patient himself superimposes images of objects by manipulating the arms of the amblyoscope. These angles are determined clinically using dissimilar, incomplete, Grade I, simultaneous macular perception slides in the major amblyoscope or other haploscopic devices. Comparison of these angles indicates the status of retinal correspondence, at least at the level of dissociation created by the amblyoscope. When the objective and subjective angles are the same, retinal correspondence is normal. When the subjective angle is 0 and the objective angle either plus (base out) or minus (base in), harmonious anomalous retinal correspondence is present. When the subjective angle is less than the objective angle but other than 0, nonharmonious anomalous retinal correspondence is present. If no subjective angle can be determined with Grade I slides, first-degree fusion is absent. First-degree fusion and normal retinal correspondence are favorable but by no means certain indications that a functional result with fusion may be obtained from surgery.

Second-degree fusion

Range of fusion. If a subjective angle is found with appropriate slides, Grade II fusion targets are inserted into the arms of the major amblyoscope and the patient's fusional amplitudes are determined. Grade II fusion slides are similar in their overall outline, differing only in detail. These differences serve as checkpoints. With Grade II targets in the amblyoscope, the arms are first shifted outward (exo) and then inward (eso). Fusional amplitudes are an expression of the patient's ability to keep the images one and and therefore fused by either diverging or converging his eyes as the arms of the amblyscope are shifted outward and inward. Fusional divergence is usually tested before fusional convergence. A "make" and "break" point for each is recorded; for example: −6 to −4; +40 to +28. This means that the patient experienced diplopia when the arms got to 6 Δ exodeviation, but he was able to refuse the images while 4 Δ exodeviated; fusion was held to 40 Δ of convergence before diplopia appeared and the doubled images were refused at convergence of 28 Δ. The presence of second-degree fusion indicates that a functional result with fusion and fusion amplitudes should be obtainable with proper surgery. Such patients should usually be slightly overcorrected to obtain the best and most lasting results from surgery.

Suppression. If no subjective angle is determined and therefore no Grade I fusion is present, suppression is recorded.

Superimposition. Superimposition is checked if the patient is able to appreciate the Grade I fusion slides simultaneously.

Fusional amplitudes. If the patient has amplitudes and therefore Grade II fusion, fusion is checked and the amplitudes are recorded.

Stereoacuity. The Titmus vectograph is used to test stereoacuity and findings are recorded as fly, A, B, C animals, and the fraction of the nine dots that the patient can appreciate. Stereopsis is rarely found in manifest strabismus of sufficient size to warrant surgery, but it may be quite good in intermittent deviations or small angle manifest strabismus with peripheral fusion.

Worth four dot testing. Worth four dot testing is done at variable near distances and at 20 feet. Results of this testing are recorded as *fusion, diplopia, alternation,* or *suppression of one eye.* In many instances, patients with small angle esotropia and peripheral fusion will fuse the four lights at near but not at distance. Some gross estimation of the size of the functional scotoma that occurs during binocular vision in patients with small angle strabismus can be made by determining how far the four lights must be removed from the patient before suppression occurs. The retinal image created by the four lights becomes smaller as the lights recede from the patient. The Worth four dot test may also be considered a gross color vision test and retinal correspondence test. If four lights in proper alignment are seen in the presence of a manifest strabismus , harmonious anomalous retinal correspondence may be inferred.

Bagolini striated glasses. Bagolini glasses placed in a trial frame with their axes at 135° OD and 45° OS may be used to determine retinal correspondence in casual seeing. Nearly all strabismic patients respond that they see diagonal lines intersecting at the light (harmonious anomalous retinal correspondence) or that they see one diagonal line with or without an incomplete second diagonal line (complete or partial suppression of one eye). Results of this test do not influence surgical judgment.

Afterimage test. The afterimage test is used to determine retinal correspondence in extreme dissociation. Anomalous retinal correspondence occurring on the afterimage test indicates a deep sensory anomaly and indicates that a functional result with fusion is unlikely to result from surgery.

Fixation. Fixation behavior is determined with the Visuscope or with an ophthalmoscope that contains a fixation target or that has been modified by having a tiny hole drilled in the red free filter. Fixation behavior is mapped out directly on the chart. Amblyopia with peripheral eccentric fixation indicates the possibility of a significant overcorrection of an esodeviation even when moderate amounts of surgery are done.

Sensory testing is useful both preoperatively and postoperatively. The closer to normal the sensory findings are preoperatively, the more active the surgeon should be in attempting a slight surgical overcorrection that would lead to a functional fusion result from surgery. Postoperative sensory testing serves as a check on surgical results from the functional standpoint and serves as a guide to further nonsurgical treatment, which should be pursued vigorously if an undercorrection has been obtained in a potentially fusing patient.

PRISM COVER TESTING

Alternate prism and cover testing is carried out to measure the maximum deviation. This testing is done at distance (20 feet) and near (13 inches), with and without glasses, while the patient views an *accommodative* target in the primary position. The use of an accommodative target is an essential part of this test because it controls the patient's accommodative convergence. Prism and cover testing is also done in approximately 30° of up and down gaze while the patient wears his full correction and views an accommodative target in the distance. If this test is done at near the patient should wear +3.00 D lenses over his distance correction. Up and down gaze is achieved by tilting the patient's head backward and forward. This maneuver uncovers an A or V pattern. A 10 Δ difference is significant for an A pattern and a 15 Δ difference is significant for a V pattern.

Other useful variations of prism and cover testing that may be done before or after the alternate prism and cover test include the following:

1. The cover-uncover test determines the presence or absence of a tropia. (If phoria is found, the phoria can be measured with alternate prism and cover testing.)

2. Lateral gaze prism and cover testing determines the presence of lateral incomitance, which is especially important in exodeviations.

3. Prism and cover testing with either eye fixing helps to determine the primary and secondary deviation.

4. Simultaneous prism and cover testing (SPC) determines the actual tropia in casual seeing in patients where a tropia and phoria coexist (monofixational esophoria, monofixation syndrome, microstrabismus, or small angle tropia with peripheral fusion).

5. The Hirschberg test compares the location of the corneal light reflexes relative to the central pupillary axes and is done when patient cooperation is poor.

For each millimeter of displacement of the corneal light reflex in the nonfixing eye, approximately 15 Δ of deviation exists.

6. The Krimsky test determines the amount of prism that must be placed before the fixing eye to center the corneal light reflex in the pupil of the nonfixing eye. It is used when the patient has such poor vision in one eye that fixation is not taken up well with that eye during prism and cover testing.

7. Cardinal position prism and cover testing with either eye fixing in the nine diagnostic positions of gaze is done in cases of muscle palsy, particularly vertical muscle palsy.

8. Dissociated vertical deviation (alternating sursumduction) is noted with cover-uncover testing and is recorded as +1 (±5 Δ) to +4 (±25 Δ).

9. Red lens and Maddox rod tests are useful in cases of small angle vertical and/or horizontal strabismus with symptomatic diplopia.

10. The double Maddox rod test is useful in diagnosis of cyclodeviations.

11. The 4 Δ base-out prism test may be used to uncover a scotoma in the macula of the one eye in patients with microtropia.

12. The Hess, Lancaster, or Lees screen may be used to plot directly the deviation in a strabismic patient who is cooperative.

REFRACTION

A cycloplegic refraction is done using 0.5% atropine solution (1 drop) or 1% atropine ointment (¼-inch strip) in each eye for 3 days prior to the day of examination. When drops are used, the atropine may also be applied on the day of the examination. Careful instructions are given to the parents to avoid overdosage. This includes using no more medicine than prescribed and holding a finger over the puncta for a few seconds after drops are instilled to reduce the possibility of significant systemic absorption of the drug. Use of atropine is usually restricted to preschool-age children. Two drops of 1% cyclopentolate (Cyclogyl) has, in my experience, provided adequate cycloplegia after 30 minutes in most school-age children. One drop of 10% phenylephrine (Neo-Synephrine) should be used in addition to the cyclopentolate in patients with dark irides. In children under 1 year of age, 0.5% cyclopentolate drops are used. In esodeviations particularly, the full hyperopia must be elicited. Hyperopia as low as +1.50 D should receive a trial treatment with glasses in patients with esotropia *beginning* after 1 year of age. Echothiophate iodide (Phospholine Iodide) drops (0.03% to 0.125%, one drop in each eye each morning for 3 weeks) may help to determine what effect the hyperopia (accommodative effort) has on the esodeviation, but because anticholinesterase drops only reduce the effective AC/A and do not eliminate the need for accommodation, they are not a true substitute for glasses.

FUNDUS EXAMINATION

Examination of the retina may be carried out using a portable indirect ophthalmoscope. It is a relatively simple matter to see the entire retina posterior to the equator in a squirming infant using the indirect ophthalmoscope. This examination to rule out pathology in the posterior pole is an essential part of the evaluation of every strabismus patient.

BIOMICROSCOPIC EXAMINATION

Examination of the anterior segment should be done on all cooperative patients, particularly when echothiophate iodide is used, because of the possibility of iris cysts and to confirm continued clarity of the lens.

DIAGNOSIS

When sufficient historical data and motility measurements have been recorded, a diagnosis is made. This diagnosis can be made in most cases after the initial examination, but repeated measurements at one or more subsequent visits should be done before a final diagnosis is made and a specific surgical treatment plan decided upon. The diagnosis should include all facets of the strabismus problem, including notation of some or all of the following:

1. Etiology
2. Direction of deviation (eso, exo, hyper)
3. Concomitance
4. Fixation behavior
5. Vision
6. Accommodative factors
7. AC/A
8. Manifest or latent
9. A or V pattern
10. Forced ductions
11. Saccadic velocity
12. Muscle force

TREATMENT

A plan for surgical treatment should be placed on the patient's record at the time the patient is scheduled for surgery. In most instances the specific muscles to be operated upon and the direction and amount they are to be weakened, strengthened, or shifted will be known. This plan is not influenced by the alignment of the eyes in the operating room after surgical anesthesia has been obtained. However, in those patients with restricted motility, and particularly in those who have been operated upon previously, the type and amount of surgery can often be decided upon only after performing forced ductions while the patient is asleep and after assessing the state of the muscles and associated restrictive fascia at the time of surgery.

As a rule, all previously operated muscles that are being considered for surgery should be identified before any strengthening, weakening, or transfer procedures are done. In such cases findings at the time of surgery may alter the surgical plan. For example, in a patient with secondary exotropia occurring after recession of the medial rectus and resection of the lateral rectus for esotropia, the lateral rectus would require weakening and the medial rectus strengthening. If treated like a new case, the lateral rectus would be weakened first and then the medial rectus strengthened. This follows the rule of doing the recession first in recession-resection procedures. However, in secondary cases where two muscles will be operated upon, the muscle to be strengthened is isolated first and tagged with a 4-0 silk suture. This is essential for two reasons: (1) to determine

209

what effect freeing of adhesions will have on the forced ductions, and (2) to determine whether a muscle is indeed present. The condition of the muscle to be strengthened may influence the amount of weakening that should be done on the antagonist or may indicate that a muscle transfer should be done. Esotropia occurring after surgery for exotropia and with limited forced (and voluntary) abduction may be treated with recession of a tight medial rectus alone, provided muscle force generation of the lateral rectus is adequate.

As mentioned previously, nonsurgical treatment will not be discussed in this text. All appropriate nonsurgical treatment including glasses, prisms, anticholinesterase, occlusion, orthoptics, and the like should be carried out in appropriate cases before embarking upon surgery.

Step 2: Results to be expected from surgery

HORIZONTAL RECTUS SURGERY FOR ESOTROPIA

Single muscle procedures for esotropia

In general, surgery done on a single horizontal rectus muscle as primary treatment of esotropia is to be avoided. However, Chamberlain found that when indicated in patients with small angle esotropia and fusion potential, a single medial rectus recession of 4 mm will produce approximately 13 Δ of correction. It should be emphasized that one must have a good reason for doing a single medial rectus recession. This reason is usually that the patient has diplopia and/or asthenopia and displays good potential for bifoveal fusion. The majority of individuals who have a small angle esotropia with an angle sufficiently small to be corrected by a single medial rectus recession have *peripheral* fusion and harmonious anomalous retinal correspondence and are included in the monofixation syndrome. Such patients are cosmetically acceptable and should not be operated. A single medial rectus recession done out of fear of producing an overcorrection is usually a manifestation of trepidation on the part of the overcautious surgeon. Single medial rectus recession for patients with limitation of motility such as Duane's syndrome is discussed elsewhere.

Resection of a single lateral rectus muscle for esotropia is even less effective than recession of a single medial rectus muscle and is even less likely to be indicated.

Two muscle surgery for esotropia

Bimedial rectus recession. A minimal bimedial rectus recession of 2.5 mm reduces an esodeviation approximately 15 Δ to 20 Δ. A maximum bimedial rectus recession of 5.0 to 6.0 mm results in approximately 50 Δ less esodeviation postoperatively. Slightly more effect may be obtained in infants but definitely less effect is produced in adults. In Indiana University Clinic a bimedial rectus recession has in the past been done for children who have the following characteristics:

1. Esotropia of 40 Δ or less
2. Equal vision
3. Esotropia greater at near (high AC/A)
4. Excess adduction

A bimedial rectus recession may also be done in patients with an A or V pattern esotropia of 40 Δ or less with or without oblique dysfunction. When no

210

oblique dysfunction is present the medial rectus muscles are shifted vertically toward the closed end of the pattern. The recessed medial rectus muscles are shifted upward for an A pattern and downward for a V pattern. In patients with less than 40 Δ of esotropia and a V pattern with inferior oblique overaction, a bimedial rectus recession and bilateral inferior oblique myectomy may be done in order to divide the amount of surgery equally, hoping for more symmetrical results. The disire for symmetry, however, is not a consistent indication for doing a bimedial rectus recession.

"En bloc" bimedial rectus recession. For the past year in the ocular motility clinic of the Indiana University Medical Center, all congenital estropia patients undergoing surgery have received a bimedial rectus recession. Each medial rectus was recessed according to the usual amount, but for children under 1 year of age 5.0 mm was added and the muscle was recessed measuring from the limbus. In children over age 1 year, 5.5 mm was added and the muscle was recessed measuring from the limbus. For example, if a 4.0 mm bimedial rectus recession was to be done in a child 2 years of age, the muscles were reattached 9.5 mm from the limbus. In addition to measuring from the limbus, a conjunctival recession of between 3 and 6 mm was carried out on each patient. Final results of this study are not available at this time. However, preliminary results indicate that the amount of correction obtained from an en bloc recession is greater in number of prism diopters corrected per millimeter of surgery, and, in addition to this, when measuring from the limbus, more millimeters of surgery are done. The average medial rectus insertion in sixty-six consecutive congenital esotropia patients was 4.3 mm from the limbus.

Bilateral lateral rectus resection. Bilateral lateral rectus resection is a procedure I seldom do. However, this procedure is frequently employed by those who routinely do a bimedial rectus recession as an initial procedure for large angle, congenital esotropia without conjunctival recession. As a rule, a bilateral strengthening procedure of the rectus muscles without recession of their antagonists is less effective at reducing the angle of strabismus than a bilateral weakening procedure without strengthening of the antagonists, and it is considerably less effective than the same resection combined with a recession of the antagonist done at the same procedure. Two situations that indicate bilateral lateral rectus resection are divergence insufficiency (paralysis) and residual esotropia in a patient who has had a bimedial rectus recession. Approximately 20 Δ of esodeviation is corrected with a minimal 5.0-mm bilateral lateral rectus resection and up to 35 Δ to 40 Δ of esotropia can be corrected with a maximum 9.0-mm to 10.0+-mm bilateral lateral rectus resection.

Recession of the medial rectus–resection of the lateral rectus. A minimum recession-resection procedure for esotropia is a 2.5-mm medial rectus recession and a 5.0-mm lateral rectus resection. This could be expected to correct 20 Δ to 25 Δ of esotropia. A maximum recession-resection procedure in a child less than age 1 year of 5.0-mm medial rectus recession and 9.0-mm lateral rectus resection and in a child over age 3 years of 5.5-mm medial rectus recession and 10.0+-mm lateral rectus resection, corrects up to 50 Δ of esotropia. Increasing the minimum numbers or decreasing the maximum numbers can be carried out for deviations between 20 Δ and 50 Δ of esotropia and for children falling between the ages of 1 and 3 years.

211

The amount of surgery may be divided between the medial and lateral rectus according to findings on ductions and versions as well as upon differences between distance and near measurements. If excess adduction and/or greater deviation at near is found, more emphasis is placed on the medial rectus recession. If deficient abduction and/or greater deviation in the distance is present, more emphasis is placed on the lateral rectus resection. This represents the symmetrizing effect of the recession-resection procedure.

Three muscle surgery for esotropia

Bimedial rectus recession and lateral rectus resection. When more than 50 Δ of esotropia must be corrected, surgery usually should be done on three muscles.* A maximum three muscle procedure will correct up to 75 Δ of esotropia. This maximum procedure consists of a bimedial 4.5-mm medial rectus recession and 9.0-mm resection of one lateral rectus (less than 1 year) and a bimedial 5.0-mm rectus recession and 10.0+-mm resection of one lateral rectus (over 3 years). Deviations between 50 Δ and 75 Δ are corrected by reducing maximum three muscle surgery by 0.5 to 1.0 mm per muscle. Three muscle surgery for esotropia has been criticized on the grounds that after such surgery only one unoperated muscle remains. Under these conditions, it has been said that it is more difficult to correct any residual esodeviation that might remain. However, residual esotropia in this type of case can be treated effectively with a marginal myotomy of a previously recessed medial rectus muscle combined with a resection of the unoperated lateral rectus muscle. This technique has in my experience been very effective as treatment for residual esotropia after prior three muscle surgery.

Four muscle surgery for esotropia

Bimedial rectus recession–bilateral lateral rectus resection. Esotropia greater than 75 Δ may be treated surgically with a bilateral recession-resection procedure. This four muscle procedure should be employed with discretion and is not often indicated. Four muscle surgery should not be done in infants. However, certain adults and older children with esodeviations of between 75 Δ and 100 Δ, particularly with limitation of forced abduction, Möbius syndrome, for example, can benefit from a bimedial 5.0-mm rectus recession and a 10.0-mm bilateral lateral rectus resection. Four muscle surgery should be limited to these maximum numbers, if it is to be done at all.

HORIZONTAL RECTUS SURGERY FOR EXOTROPIA
Single muscle surgery for exotropia

A single lateral rectus recession or a single medial rectus resection for treatment of exotropia is rarely indicated. However, certain patients who have a very small incomitant exotropia and who have fusion potential can be helped by such a procedure. These patients are rare, since their condition is usually caused in the first place by insufficient initial surgery in which only one lateral rectus muscle was recessed. In such a case, either the medial rectus should be resected or the lateral rectus recessed to produce the most nearly comitant end result. The

---

*Except in congenital esotropia where a maximum "en bloc" recession is carried out in all patients with a deviation greater than 50 Δ.

finding on versions and ductions, as well as prism and cover measurements in the lateral versions, indicate what should be done to achieve comitance. No more than 15 Δ of deviation can be corrected with single muscle surgery for exotropia.

Two muscle surgery for exotropia

Bilateral lateral rectus recession. A minimum bilateral lateral rectus recession of 5.0 mm will correct approximately 20 Δ to 25 Δ of exotropia. A maximum bilateral lateral rectus recession of 8.0+ mm can correct up to 50 Δ of exotropia. In Indiana University Clinic, a bilateral lateral rectus recession is done only in patients with true divergence excess exotropia (distance exotropia greater than near exotropia), which may be manifest or latent.

Bimedial rectus resection. "Strengthening" and "weakening" procedures of the extraocular muscles in the main improve ocular alignment while maintaining or creating comitance. On the other hand such extraocular muscle surgery *does not* ordinarily influence vergences. In spite of this, certain patients demonstrating "intractable" convergence insufficiency not helped by near point exercises or other orthoptic treatment may be helped with a bimedial rectus resection. A 6.0- to 8.0-mm bimedial rectus resection can be considered reasonable treatment for a convergence insufficiency measuring between 12 Δ and 25 Δ of exotropia at near with a remote near point of convergence.

Intermittent exotropia persisting after bilateral lateral rectus recession can also be treated with a bimedial rectus resection. In such a case, a minimum 5.0-mm bimedial rectus resection can correct approximately 20 Δ of exotropia. A maximum, 10.0+-mm bilateral medial rectus resection can correct up to 40 Δ of exotropia.

Lateral rectus recession–medial rectus resection. A minimum recession-resection procedure for exotropia is 5.0-mm lateral rectus recession and 5.0-mm medial rectus resection. This will correct approximately 20 Δ to 25 Δ of exotropia and produce about the same reduction in the exotropia in the distance and at near. A maximum recession-resection procedure for exotropia is 8.0-mm lateral rectus recession* and 10.0+-mm medial rectus resection. This would be expected to correct up to 50 Δ of exotropia. Since the majority of exotropic patients in my experience are basic exotropia (same exotropia distance and near) or simulated divergence excess exotropia (near exotropia equal to or nearly equal to distance exotropia after several hours occlusion of one eye), a recession-resection procedure is the most common exotropia procedure I use. In exotropia my experience has been that a recession-resection procedure is the most effective and predictable way to alter the alignment of the eyes in order to produce cosmetic as well as functional improvement. Surgically induced incomitance is infrequent, and when it does occur is not usually significant.

Three muscle surgery for exotropia

A maximum bilateral lateral rectus recession of 8.0+ mm combined with a maximum medial rectus resection of 10.0+ mm in one eye will correct up to 75 Δ of exotropia. To correct deviations between 50 Δ and 75 Δ maximum, three muscle surgery is reduced by 0.5 to 1.0 mm per muscle.

---

*Some surgeons consider a 10.0-mm lateral rectus recession as a reasonable maximum.

For XT less than 20 Δ eg: — 18-20 Δ do Subminimal R&R eg:- 4 mm Recess & 4 mm Resect

✗. In alternating XT (c̄ no preference for any eye) do R&R in OD in this country so that there is no limitation of Lat. gaze in OS. since there is a left handed traffic.

213

Four muscle surgery for exotropia

A maximum 8.0+-mm bilateral lateral rectus recession combined with a maximum 10.0+-mm bimedial rectus recession will correct 90 Δ to 100 Δ of exotropia. If four muscle surgery is indicated for exotropia, maximum amounts should be done.

VERTICAL RECTUS SURGERY

Single muscle surgery done on the vertical rectus muscles can be effective and predictable. This is in contrast to single muscle surgery done on the horizontal rectus muscles, which is not. A minimum 2.5-mm recession or resection of either the superior or inferior rectus will produce approximately 8 Δ of reduction of the deviation in the primary position and slightly more in the field of action of the muscle. A usual maximum 5.0-mm recession or resection of a vertically acting rectus muscle will produce up to 15 Δ of reduction of the deviation in the primary position and slightly more in the field of action of the muscle. A combined recession-resection of the vertical rectus corrects with minimum "numbers" 15 Δ and with maximum "numbers" 25 Δ to 30 Δ in the primary position. The normal maximums for recession and resection of the inferior rectus can be exceeded in patients who demonstrate restriction on testing with forced ductions from such causes as thyroid myopathy, old blowout fractures, fibrosis syndrome, or prior surgery. In such selected cases, the inferior rectus can be resected up to 10.0 mm and recessed up to 10.0 mm or even more.

I have done a "guarded free tenotomy" of the inferior rectus in patients with severe thyroid myopathy affecting the inferior rectus and have produced marked improvement in motility with only moderate ptosis of the lower lid resulting in 2.0 to 3.0 mm widening of the palpebral fissure. More recently these large recessions have been carried out using an adjustable suture. In two patients with marked hyperdeviation after repeated muscle surgery, we have done 9.0-mm resections of the inferior rectus without causing significant narrowing of the palpebral fissure. It should be emphasized, however, that patients should be selected very carefully before exceeding the usual limits of recession and resection on the inferior rectus. The superior rectus should not ordinarily be resected more than 5.0 mm. Ptosis involving the upper lid is easier to produce, harder to avoid, and cosmetically more objectionable than similar displacement of the lower lid. With careful dissection of the intermuscular membrane and taking care not to cut the superior oblique tendon, the superior rectus may be recessed 5.0 or 6.0 mm or more without causing retraction of the upper lid.

SURGERY OF THE OBLIQUE MUSCLES

Superior oblique weakening. Tenotomy of the superior oblique muscle produces approximately 10 Δ to 15 Δ reduction in the hypodeviation in the primary position and slightly greater reduction in the field of action of the muscle. This procedure may be graded somewhat by shifting the site of the tenotomy closer to the insertion for less effect or closer to the trochlea for more effect, or it may be graded with a guarded suture. If a tenectomy is done, the degree of weakening of the superior oblique is probably not affected by the amount of tendon removed but rather by the proximity of the nasal extent of the tenectomy to the trochlea. The fascia in the vicinity of the superior oblique tendon should be left intact when doing a superior oblique tenotomy to achieve more predictable results. In practice, unilateral superior oblique weakening is seldom done. Bilateral superior oblique weakening is more common and is discussed in the section on surgery for A and V patterns.

Superior oblique strengthening. Strengthening of the superior oblique by a tuck at its insertion produces up to 15 Δ reduction in the hyperdeviation in the primary position and 25 Δ reduction in the hyperdeviation in the field of action of this muscle. The amount of the superior oblique that should be tucked depends upon how lax or redundant the tendon is at the time of the surgery. During surgery, the tendon is brought up into the tucker until the tendon feels taut and at this point the tuck is secured. For smaller deviations, tension is relaxed on the tendon by reducing the tuck by 2.0 mm before securing the tuck. The size of the tuck may vary from 8.0 to 20.0 mm or more.

Sagittalization of the superior oblique. The intorting power of the superior oblique may be increased by moving all or part of the effective insertion anteriorly. A tucking procedure in my hands improves the torsional deviation at the same time as improving the vertical deviation. However, when a large torsional deviation of 10° to 15° is present in a patient who has a small vertical deviation, a sagittalization procedure is a useful surgical tool.

Inferior oblique weakening. Weakening of the inferior oblique muscle produces 10 Δ to 15 Δ reduction in hyperdeviation in the primary position and slightly more in the field of action of this muscle. Inferior oblique weakening procedures are not ordinarily graded. When a recession is done it is usually 8.0 mm. Disinsertion merely frees the muscle from its insertion. With a myectomy, a 5.0-mm piece of muscle is excised below the inferior border of the lateral rectus in the inferior temporal quadrant. Marginal or incomplete myotomies or disinsertions of the inferior oblique are not effective and should not be done.

Inferior oblique strengthening. Strengthening procedures of the inferior oblique muscle have, in my hands, proved unsatisfactory for treating vertical misalignment, so no figures can be given for expected correction. If a tuck is done, no less than 10.0 mm of the muscle should be included. If resection and advancement are done approximately 5.0 mm of the muscle should be resected and the muscle should be advanced 5.0 mm.

SURGERY FOR VERTICALLY INCOMITANT HORIZONTAL STRABISMUS (A AND V PATTERNS)

When surgery is done to treat vertical incomitance, a fixed amount of surgery is performed. This is accomplished by shifting the horizontal rectus insertions upward or downward or by weakening overacting oblique muscles.

Bilateral inferior oblique myectomy for treating a V pattern produces on the average 20 Δ less exotropia or more esotropia in up gaze. Bilateral superior oblique tenotomy for treating an A pattern produces from 7 Δ to 70 Δ less exodeviation or more esodeviation in down gaze. The average change of alignment in down gaze after bilateral superior oblique tenectomy is 32 Δ. With a fixed amount of either inferior or superior oblique weakening, more effect is produced

215

If in an A pattern c̄ XT of ~~more~~ less than 20Δ XT → Knapp says no need for correction for XT, S.O. tenotomy will correct it. [Practically this is not true, it needs a separate surgery for correction of XT along c̄ S.O. tenotomy.]

in large A or V patterns and less effect in small A or V patterns. This represents a type of built-in safety factor for this surgery.

The horizontal rectus muscles may be shifted one-half to one muscle width upward or downward. This produces 20 Δ to 25 Δ change in the A or V pattern. The medial rectus muscles are always moved in the direction of the apex of the A or V, and the lateral rectus muscles are always moved toward the open end of the A or V. Vertical shift of the horizontal rectus muscles may be done with symmetrical surgery (bilateral recession or resections) or when a recession-resection is done. The horizontal rectus muscles also may be moved vertically without recession or resection in cases of A or V pattern without oblique dysfunction and where no horizontal deviation is present in the primary position.

I have had no experience with horizontal shift of the vertical rectus for treatment of A and V patterns. According to those surgeons who have used this procedure, lateral shift of the inferior rectus muscles in V esotropia without a deviation in the primary position and without oblique muscle dysfunction has proved useful.

THE FADEN OPERATION *Indi. on pg. (135)*

The Faden operation (translated: suture operation) or posterior fixation suture has gained great popularity in Europe after its introduction by Cüppers. This procedure is now being used with increased frequency in the United States and Canada. The procedure has been used mostly in treating the so-called block nystagmus syndrome, dissociated vertical deviation, and nystagmus. The essence of the procedure is that it weakens a muscle and its field of action but does not affect the primary position deviation or the action of the antagonist of the operated muscle. In cases of esotropia with block nystagmus, the Faden operation is combined with appropriate recession of the medial rectus muscles. Results of this surgery are good, according to some, but, when the Faden operation is combined with a recession, it is difficult to know which part of the procedure is affecting the deviation. I have had some success in treating dissociated vertical deviation with the Faden operation, but it is not possible for me to make a final, personal judgment regarding the effectiveness of this procedure.

Summary of steps 1 and 2 in the design of strabismus surgery

When an accurate workup has been completed and a pertinent history recorded, a surgeon should possess sufficient knowledge of the patient and his strabismus problem to have certain goals for the patient in mind. He should also have certain expectations with regard to the results he can achieve from surgery in that particular patient. Added to this the surgeon knows approximately how much change in ocular alignment he can expect to produce with those muscle strengthening and weakening procedures appropriate for the patient. It is the union of these two factors (measurements and results to be expected from surgery) that enables the surgeon to design each surgical procedure specifically for each individual patient. This combination of measurement with usual results is made more sensitive by the application of certain rules that give hints as to how certain types of patient may be expected to respond to strabismus surgery.

Here it should be reemphasized that orthoptic, optical, and certain pharma-

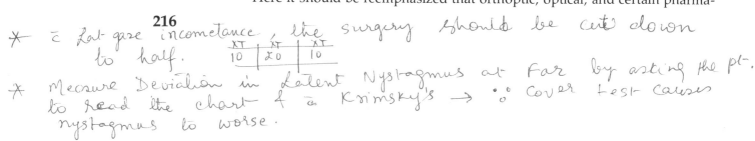

216

* c̄ Lat gaze incomelance, the surgery should be cut down to half.
| | XT | XT | XT |
| | 10 | 20 | 10 |

* Measure Deviation in Latent Nystagmus at Far by asking the pt. to read the chart f̄ c̄ Krimsky's → ∴ Cover test causes nystagmus to worse.

cologic therapy is superior to surgical therapy for strabismus, provided these nonsurgical methods result in comfortable fusion and the accompanying acceptable appearance. Surgery should be done only to reduce a cosmetically objectionable tropia or to enable comfortable fusion in patients who cannot be helped by nonsurgical means.

Step 3: How to apply surgical options

The third component in the design of the surgical procedure joins step 1 (the workup) and step 2 (surgical options). The following aphorisms may be applied to help produce this happy and successful union between the patient and his surgical "numbers."

1. If fusion has ever been present a functional cure with fusion may be expected. A slight overcorrection helps obtain such a functional cure.

2. If no fusion potential is present a slight undercorrection is more likely to produce a stable, cosmetically acceptable, small angle residual deviation.

3. The surgeon should aim at a cure with his first surgery provided there are sufficient muscles to operate upon without causing complications such as anterior segment necrosis.

4. The surgeon should strive toward judicious boldness and not be excessively fearful of producing an overcorrection.

5. If a surgeon is doing the proper amount of surgery, he should expect some overcorrections and not produce an excessive number of undercorrections with regard to intended results. For example, if a surgeon aims at a 5 Δ undercorrection, a patient who is ortho in the early postoperative period represents a relative overcorrection.

6. More effect is produced per millimeter of recession or resection by strabismus surgery done in a child or in a patient with a small eye; less effect is produced by strabismus surgery done in an adult or in a patient with a large eye.

7. More effect is gained from strabismus surgery done on a recent deviation than on a long-standing deviation.

8. Surgery done for a small deviation (±25 Δ) produces less effect per millimeter of surgery than that done for a larger deviation (±50 Δ).

9. In patients with cerebral palsy and strabismus, the more cephalad the neurologic involvement, the longer surgery should be delayed. Patients with only limb involvement in which the cranial nerves are spared may be treated as an otherwise normal strabismic child.

10. In partially accommodative esotropia, only the nonaccommodative part of the deviation should be treated surgically.

11. One 4.0-mm medial rectus recession corrects approximately 13 Δ of esotropia.

12. Conjunctival recession done routinely with bimedial recession for congenital esotropia increases the number of prism diopters of effect per millimeter of surgery by about 25%.

13. A minimal recession-resection for either esotropia or exotropia produces approximately 25 Δ reduction in the esodeviation or exodeviation.

14. A maximum recession-resection procedure for either esotropia or exo-

217

See other of Stanbian page 116

Also See page 200.

See page 200

Secondary XT → following overcorrection of previous ET →

(1) if marked limitation of passive adduction of OS → suggests tight LR Recession or marginal myotomies of L.R. indicated.

(2) Unrestricted passive adduction of OS but defective active adduction suggests Re of MR was too extensive. The MR should be advanced & resected

tropia produces approximately 50 Δ reduction in the esodeviation or exodeviation.

15. Three muscle surgery for esotropia or exotropia may be required for deviations greater than 50 Δ but less than 75 Δ.

16. Four muscle surgery for either esotropia or exotropia may be required for deviations greater than 75 Δ but is done rarely in children.

17. Esodeviations or exodeviations greater than 50 Δ in a patient with very poor vision in one eye should be treated with a supermaximal recession-resection of one eye to avoid surgery on the better eye.

18. Surgery for esotropia in a hyperkinetic child produces less effect than the same amount of surgery done in a normal child.

19. Residual esotropia after a bimedial rectus recession that had been done several years before should be treated with a marginal myotomy of one previously recessed medial rectus and a resection of one lateral rectus if the deviation is ±25 Δ. This procedure should be done bilaterally if the deviation is ±50 Δ. For deviations between 30 Δ and 50 Δ a resection of the lateral rectus alone may be done in the second eye.

20. Residual esotropia occurring weeks to months after a bimedial rectus recession should be treated with a bilateral lateral rectus resection or a rerecession of the already recessed medial rectus muscles.

21. A double 80% marginal myotomy combined with a resection of the antagonist produces the same weakening effect as a maximum recession of that muscle, provided it is combined with a resection of the antagonist. A marginal myotomy done without resection of the antagonist is not ordinarily an effective procedure. See Page 132 for Indi. of marginal myotomy.

22. A bilateral lateral rectus recession is done for exotropia less than 40 Δ that is greater in the distance with excess abduction and equal vision.

23. Exotropic patients who have lateral incomitance—that is, who have less exodeviation in lateral versions—tend to be overcorrected more easily than patients whose exodeviation is the same in the primary position as it is in lateral versions.

24. Exotropic patients who have had extensive preoperative orthoptics, especially near point of convergence exercises, are prone to large overcorrections after surgery.

25. The choice of muscles to be operated upon in the surgical treatment of intermittent exotropia is indicated by the pattern of deviation. Divergence excess exotropia is treated with bilateral lateral rectus recession; basic exotropia and simulated divergence excess exotropia are treated with a recession of the lateral rectus and a resection of the medial rectus.

26. The timing of surgery for intermittent exotropia is dictated by how often the deviation is manifested.

27. Once surgery has been decided upon for a patient with intermittent exotropia, the amount of surgery is dictated solely by the angle of the deviation and is in no way influenced by the amount of time deviation is either latent or manifest.

28. Bilateral inferior oblique myectomy produces 20 Δ less exotropia or more esotropia in up gaze with no significant change of the alignment in the primary position or in down gaze.

218

Miotics — Indi —
- Small angle ET after Surgery
- to R/o Acc component in ET preop
- High Ac/A ratio
- Surgically over corrected Intermittent XT.

Variable ET → do Surgery for minimum amount of deviation after several exams.

Residual ET treated earlier → by bimedial Recm should be treated c bilat. resection but it should be done c in 6 wks

Residual ET treated earlier Bimedial Recm → applies to ET & XT → L.R. Resect; clean scar tissue near M.R & B.S.C. & or marginal myotomy of M.R.

XT c amblyopia → overcorrect it slightly so that pt. looks good for sometime since they go XT again later.

XT usually do not have amblyopia ∴ if amblyopia + look for anisometropia or other causes of amblyopia

Variable XT - do Surgery for Maximum deviation after several exams.

See page 200

* PF's c bilat. 6th n. palsy Never fuse.
* 'V' pattern means overaction of bilat- I.O.

V ET →
V XT

— Surgical correction done for primary deviation.

29. Unequal bilateral overaction of the inferior obliques causing a V pattern should be treated with an equal weakening procedure on both inferior obliques. If only the more overacting inferior oblique is weakened, a markedly unequal overaction of the obliques, with the nonoperated muscle becoming much more overactive, will be present postoperatively.

[Handwritten left margin: Decrease in XT → not predictable]

30. Bilateral superior oblique tenotomy produces a decrease in exotropia in down gaze of between 7 Δ and 70 Δ. The average change is 32 Δ. The smaller the A, the less the change in down gaze; the more the A, the greater the change in down gaze.

[Handwritten right margin: → done in ET or XT]

31. Vertical shift of the horizontal rectus muscles for A and V patterns is done as follows: The medial rectus muscles are shifted toward the apex of the A or V, that is, up in A pattern and down in V pattern. Lateral rectus muscles are moved toward the open end of the A pattern, that is, downward in A pattern and upward in V pattern. Vertical shift of the horizontal rectus muscles (one-half to one muscle width) produces approximately 20 Δ to 25 Δ change in the A and V pattern. The greater the vertical incomitance, the more the effect.

[Handwritten left margin: ↑ ET → good prognosis c surgery if not corrected will spread to 1° position]

32. Acquired superior oblique palsy should be worked up according to the individual patient's needs, treated with prisms or patching for 6 to 9 months, and if necessary treated surgically (see Knapp's classification, Plates 13-11 and 13-12).

[Handwritten left margin: ↑ ET or A XT with diagram]

33. Bilateral superior oblique palsy frequently causes cyclotropia, which is diagnosed with the double Maddox rod test and is greater than 15°.

34. When a large horizontal deviation and a small vertical deviation exist in a patient with no fusion potential, only the horizontal deviation is treated surgically.

[Handwritten left margin: ...gical correction ...sen for the ...p of A ET.]

35. A small vertical deviation in a patient with diplopia and fusion potential may be treated with surgery and/or prisms.

36. A cosmetically unacceptable vertical deviation with or without fusion potential is treated surgically by operating upon the appropriate vertically acting muscles. The vertical rectus muscles have more effect on the deviation with the eye in abduction and the obliques have more effect on the deviation with the eye in adduction.

37. Brown's superior oblique tendon sheath syndrome is treated surgically only if a cosmetically unacceptable vertical strabismus or abnormal head position is present while the patient is fixing in the primary position.

38. "Lysis of adhesions" around an extraocular muscle is usually worthless unless it is accompanied by one or more of the following: conjunctival recession, traction suture placement, marginal myotomy, rerecession, reresection, or placement of Supramid Extra muscle sleeve or sheet.

39. Replacing tight or scarred conjunctiva to its preoperative position can nullify the results of otherwise successful strabismus surgery.

40. When there is doubt about the possibility of whether restricted motility could be caused by scarred conjunctiva, a conjunctival recession should be done, leaving bare sclera.

41. Traction sutures should be anchored securely in sclera or placed in the horizontal rectus insertions to avoid unnecessary contact with the cornea. They should be left in place 5 to 7 days, watched carefully, and fix the eye in the duction opposite the restriction several degrees past the midline.

[Handwritten marginal notes:]

XT c̄ DVD - 2 ways to Rx
① DO Foden 4 Reem SR - I stage
    Rx XT — II nd stage
Recession of S·R will ↑ XT
(vertical recti are adductors)
② I.R. Resection → will cure
    DVD & XT.

42. The cosmetic improvement of straight eyes after surgery is compromised when red unsightly scars remain in the conjunctiva. One should always attempt to retain a normal, white conjunctiva postoperatively.

43. Manifest dissociated vertical deviation (alternating sursumduction) may be treated surgically by resecting one or both inferior rectus muscles, or by recessing one or both superior rectus muscles, combined with weakening one or both oblique muscles, or by a Faden operation (posterior fixation suture) of one or both superior rectus muscles.

Each surgeon should establish his own personal set of guidelines for strabismus surgery and should delete from this list those aphorisms that do not apply to his experience.

CASE REPORTS
Case 1

This patient had congenital esotropia with cross fixation. The opportunity to see such patients depends upon the parents' and/or attending physician's awareness that esotropia in an infant should be evaluated by an ophthalmologist as soon as the esodeviation is noted. Regardless of one's attitude toward early surgery, infantile esotropia should be evaluated immediately because of the possibility that retinoblastoma, a brain tumor, or some other organic lesion may be the cause of the esodeviation.

In patients such as this with free alternation and cross fixation, the status of the lateral rectus muscles must be determined. This can be done by using the Doll's head technique, which is accomplished by gently but abruptly rotating the patient's head in one direction and then the other while watching for passive abduction of each eye. It is not necessary for the eyes to abduct fully. If they go beyond the midline on the Doll's head maneuver, lateral rectus function is confirmed. If abduction is not observed alternate patching with observation by the parents at home should be carried out.

Screen comitance testing can be done in a patient of this age only with great difficulty. For this reason it is possible that overaction of the obliques may be overlooked. Many children under 1 year of age who have surgery for congenital esotropia are later found to have overaction of one or both inferior oblique muscles.

The deviation in an infant can be evaluated with more or less difficulty and accuracy, depending upon the examiner's experience and patience with children. Alternate cover testing is usually quite difficult, so Krimsky or Hirschberg determination must often be resorted to.

The diagnosis of congenital esotropia with cross fixation indicates a need for surgery. The two variables in this situation are: (1) timing of surgery and (2) type and amount of surgery. Those opposed to early surgery may wait to obtain further, hopefully more reliable measurements and may put off surgery until age 1 or 2 years or even later. Those who favor early surgery would operate immediately. At the present time the matter is unsettled as to whether early surgery produces better functional results. There are those who very emphatically say "yes" and those who equally as emphatically say "no."

Without taking sides on the issue of whether better functional results are ob-

220

AGE ONSET 2 MO.	HX: BW 7# 3oz., Present wt. 16#., No fam. HX strabismus, General health OK, sits up, milestones OK.	AGE NOW 6 MO.

GLASSES (NONE /)
Atropine retinoscopy
OD +1.50
OS +1.50
ADD

	OCCLUSION	ORTHOPTICS	SURGERY
	NO	NO	NO

VISION	"E" GAME	LINEAR "E"	LETTER CHT.	PIN HOLE	OTHER
OD	/	APPEARS TO SEE WELL WITH EITHER EYE		/	/
OS	/			/	/

FIXATION
ALT. (CROSS FIXATION)

DUCTIONS
+1 excess adduction OU
+2 limitation abduction OU
abducts OU on Doll's head

SCREEN COMITANCE

HEAD POSTURE OK

AMBLYOSCOPE	RANGE	SUPP.
OBJ. =	/ TO /	SUPERIMP.
SUB. = NA	/ TO /	FUSION

STEREO NA   WORTH NA   BAG.   A.I.

45Δ ET
↑

PRISM COVER TEST

DIST. s̄ GL. = 45Δ ET alt.

DIST. c̄ GL. =

NEAR s̄ GL. = 45Δ ET alt.

NEAR c̄ GL. =

↓
45Δ ET

NA.   NA.

FIXATION

F: Normal posterior pole
EXT: Moderate epicanthus

DIAGNOSIS
1. Congenital ET with cross fixation

TREATMENT
If measurements are the same at three visits schedule for 4.5 mm
M.R. recess – 9.0 mm L.R. resect. Decide on which eye after
performing forced ductions under anesthesia.

_____ M.D.
SIGNATURE

RETURN APPT. __Post Op_____ DATE _____

tained by early surgery, I would prefer going ahead with surgery on such a patient simply to improve his appearance. I have in the past done a 4.5-mm recession of one medial rectus and a 9.0-mm resection of the lateral rectus in the same eye. I would now recess both medial rectus muscles 10.0 mm from the limbus and recess the conjunctiva to the site of the original insertion. In either event, the philosophy would be to correct this deviation nearly fully. A reasonable expectation for good results would be to obtain a stable small or ultrasmall angle esotropia with peripheral fusion. It is very unlikely that a case such as this with true congenital esotropia would result in perfect bifoveal fusion.

If in this case the history remained the same but the angle were less, proportionally smaller amounts of surgery would be done. If the deviation were larger, such as between 50 Δ and 75 Δ, consideration would be given to doing three muscles or placing the medial recti back 11.0 mm from the limbus. Some surgeons prefer never doing more than two muscles at the initial procedure for congenital esotropia. If further surgery is needed it is done 6 to 12 weeks later. I favor attempting to correct the entire deviation at the initial procedure, which in most cases thereby lessens the need for secondary surgery.

This type of clinical picture has been labeled "nystagmus compensation syndrome." In my opinion, there is no difference between infantile esotropia with cross fixation, adduction fixation preference, and nystagmoid movements on attempted abduction and von Noorden's interpretation of nystagmus compensation syndrome in infantile esotropia. I have been able to produce straight eyes in these patients with large bimedial rectus recessions combined with conjunctival recession. It is impossible to perform a posterior fixation suture on the medial recti in these patients after sufficient recession has been carried out to treat the so-called static angle.

Case 2

This patient had a "broken down" or decompensated accommodative esotropia with a moderate hyperopia and a high AC/A ration. Cycloplegic refraction failed to uncover additional hyperopia, and a therapeutic trial of echothiophate iodide 0.06% did not enable the patient to fuse, so surgery was indicated. Both the history and the findings on the amblyoscope indicated that the patient had fusion potential, giving almost certain indication that the patient would receive a functional cure with at least peripheral fusion if adequate surgery were done.

In such a case the surgeon should attempt to produce a slight overcorrection. Such a patient must wear his full plus lens correction postoperatively, and he may also require the use of bifocals to obtain fusion at near. My choice of surgery would be a 5.0-mm medial rectus recession and 8.0-mm lateral rectus resection. The medial rectus would be recessed the maximum amount because the deviation is greater at near. Less than a maximum lateral rectus resection would be done because the deviation in the distance is only 30 Δ.

222

OCULAR MOTILITY EXAMINATION

AGE ONSET	HX: Sudden onset ET., neg.	AGE NOW
3 1/2 yrs	fam. HX, normal growth and	6 yrs

HX: Sudden onset ET., neg. fam. HX, normal growth and development, good health, 1st glasses RX'd 2 mo after ET, bifocals RX'd age 4 1/2, did not wear glasses well during past summer, now ET with and without glasses.

GLASSES (RX'd age) 4 1/2	OCCLUSION	ORTHOPTICS	SURGERY
OD +4.50 + .50 x 90	2 mo OD	NO	NO
OS +5.00 +1.00 x 90	after break-		
ADD +3.00	down		

VISION	"E" GAME	LINEAR "E"	LETTER CHT.	PIN HOLE	OTHER
OD	/	/	20/25 with glasses		/
OS	/	/	20/25 with glasses		/

FIXATION   DUCTIONS   SCREEN COMITANCE
Free alt.   +1 excess adduction
             +1 decrease abduction

HEAD POSTURE   OK

AMBLYOSCOPE	RANGE	SUPP. O
OBJ. = +30	−4 TO −2 /	SUPERIMP. ✓
SUB. = +30	+12 TO +6 /	FUSION ✓

STEREO NIL   WORTH ALT   BAG. SUPP   A.I. −

28Δ ET with glasses   PRISM COVER TEST

DIST. s̄ GL. = 50Δ ET

DIST. c̄ GL. = 30Δ ET

NEAR s̄ GL. = 65Δ ET

32Δ ET with glasses   NEAR c̄ GL. = 45Δ ET
                       +3.00 = 30Δ ET

FIXATION

Cyclo RNS
OD
OS   Plano over RX
      F: OK

DIAGNOSIS

1) "Broken down" accommodative ET, 2) High AC/A
          3) Hyperopic Astigmatism

TREATMENT

Recess M.R. 5.0 mm, Resect L.R. 8.0 mm.

_____ M.D.
                SIGNATURE

RETURN APPT. ____ Post Op ____   DATE ____

OCULAR MOTILITY EXAMINATION

PLATE 13-3

Case 3

This patient had an esotropia whose time of onset was not known. The esotropia could either have been congenital or broken down accommodative. A significant amount of farsightedness and a fairly deep amblyopia that had not responded to patching were present. Occlusion therapy in the past had been inadequate, and although attempts were made to patch well, visual acuity could not be increased to better than 20/100. The parents and child were unwilling to continue occlusion. The patient had a very definite preference for left eye fixation, and right eye ductions were as would be expected with a longstanding right esotropia. Bilateral overaction of the inferior obliques graded at 3+ was also noted. The esotropic angle was moderately large and a V pattern present.

The diagnosis was V pattern esotropia with bilateral overaction of the inferior obliques, amblyopia of the right eye, and hyperopic astigmatism. In such a patient, nonsurgical therapy has certainly been unsuccessful. This patient and her parents were very anxious for a cosmetic improvement.

Such a patient is not likely to obtain a functional cure from surgery. Therefore, attempts should be made to produce a slight undercorrection of the esotropia so that hopefully a stable, small angle, cosmetically acceptable esotropia would result. It is essential in patients such as this to keep the patient slightly esotropic so that the nasal retina in the amblyopic eye will be viewing the object of regard. A recession of 4.0 mm and a resection of 8.0 mm is indicated. The V pattern with "double hypertropia" in lateral versions is also a cosmetic problem, and bilateral inferior oblique myectomies of 5.0 mm are indicated.

In such a case a functional result is not expected and the design of surgery reflects this. The parents and the patient should also be told that a secondary (postoperative) exotropia could result. Patients with amblyopia, hyperopia, and moderate to large angles of esotropia not infrequently develop a very large overcorrection, especially if surgery results in even a slight early overcorrection. Such patients can develop a spontaneous or consecutive exotropia even without surgery.

OCULAR MOTILITY EXAMINATION

AGE ONSET	HX: Normal growth and develop-	AGE NOW
2 1/2yr?	ment except for ET, 1 sib- ling, father and paternal	9 yrs

aunt ET, glasses age 3 1/2 yrs., patched at
intervals since age 3 1/2 yrs., now large angle
ET, wants RX

GLASSES (/ /)	OCCLUSION	ORTHOPTICS	SURGERY
OD +5.25 +1.75 x 110	Total of 6 mo. in	NO	NO
OS +5.00 +2.00 x 75	past 6 1/2 yrs. but		
ADD	not well after recent trial		
	6 mo. full time patch OD 20/400 to 20/100		

VISION	"E" GAME	LINEAR "E"	LETTER CHT.	PIN HOLE	OTHER
OD	/	/	20/100	/	J#2
OS	/	/	20/20	/	J#1

FIXATION

OS - unsteady OD

HEAD POSTURE OK

DUCTIONS

2+ excess add OD
2+ decrease abd OD

SCREEN COMITANCE

3+ AIO OU

AMBLYOSCOPE	RANGE		SUPP. ✓	
OBJ. = 45	/ TO /	SUPERIMP.	0	
SUB. = NO	/ TO /	FUSION	0	

STEREO NIL   WORTH OS   BAG. SUPP   A.I.

30△ ET OD

↑
│
│
↓

70△ ET OD

PRISM COVER TEST

DIST. s̄ GL. = 55△ ET OD

DIST. c̄ GL. = 45△ ET OD

NEAR s̄ GL. = 60△ ET OD

NEAR c̄ GL. = 55△ ET OD

FIXATION
Cyclogyl 1% Retinoscopy
OD
OS   Plano over RX
F: OK - OU

DIAGNOSIS

1) Esotropia, 2) Amblyopia OD, 3) Hyperopic Astigmatism, 4) "V" pattern with bilateral overaction of inferior obliques.

TREATMENT

Recess R.M.R. 4.0 mm, Resect R.L.R. 8.0 mm - Bilat. I.O. myotomy 5.0 mm.
    * Explain to parents possibility of secondary XT

_____ M.D.
SIGNATURE

RETURN APPT. _____ Post Op _____ DATE _____

OCULAR MOTILITY EXAMINATION

PLATE 13-4

Case 4

This residual esotropia was probably caused by inadequate surgery done initially. The angle was moderate and not influenced by accommodative effort. No fusion potential was apparent, and harmonious anomalous retinal correspondence had been found. There was a limitation of abduction in the right eye and a slight overaction of the inferior obliques bilaterally. A minimal "clinically insignificant" V pattern was also present. There was some uncertainty regarding the time of onset of the strabismus, but the fact that this patient had dissociated vertical deviation (alternating sursumduction) with minimal latent nystagmus indicated that the esotropia was in all likelihood congenital and therefore the chance of gaining bifoveal fusion slight.

In such a case, forced ductions must be done and interpreted at the time of surgery. The eye with greater resistance to abduction would then be the eye chosen for surgery. The operation would consist of a double 80% marginal myotomy of the medial rectus and a 7.0-mm resection of the lateral rectus to aim for a slight undercorrection. The minimal V pattern and slight overaction of the inferior obliques do not warrant surgical attention.

If this undercorrection were seen a few weeks or months after a bimedial rectus recession for congenital esotropia, I would do a bilateral resection of the lateral rectus muscles. If the dissociated vertical deviation causes a cosmetically objectionable manifest hyperdeviation of one or both eyes, a posterior fixation suture (Faden operation) along with a 3.0- to 5.0-mm recession could be done on the offending superior rectus.

OCULAR MOTILITY EXAMINATION

AGE ONSET	HX: Normal development	AGE NOW
? Birth	except for ET, 1 sibling ET, surgery age 3 yrs. had	8 yrs.

little effect, no further surgery suggested, no diplopia.

GLASSES (RX'd /elsewhere	OCCLUSION	ORTHOPTICS	SURGERY
does not wear	alt. for 3 mos.	NO	Bimedial reces-
OD +.75	prior to sur-		sion 2.5 mm age 3
OS +.50	gery.		
ADD			

VISION	"E" GAME	LINEAR "E"	LETTER CHT.	PIN HOLE	OTHER
OD	/	/	20/20	/	J#1
OS	/	/	20/20	/	J#1

FIXATION DUCTIONS SCREEN COMITANCE

ALT

HEAD POSTURE   OK

AMBLYOSCOPE   RANGE   SUPP. ✓

OBJ. = 35Δ   /   TO   /   SUPERIMP.

SUB. = 0   /   TO   /   FUSION

STEREO NIL   WORTH ALT   BAG. X   A.I. Scars Medial Conjunctiva

30Δ ET   PRISM COVER TEST

DIST. s̄ GL. =   30Δ ET

DIST. c̄ GL. =

NEAR s̄ GL. =   2+ Alt.
sursum OU

NEAR c̄ GL. =   32Δ ET

35Δ ET

FIXATION

Cyclogyl 1% Retinoscopy
    OD +.25
    OS +.50
    F: OK

DIAGNOSIS

1) Residual Esotropia

TREATMENT

Schedule for EOM surgery - do FD under anesthesia, plan 80%
double MM - M.R. OD. Resect L.R. OD 7.0 mm.

_____ M.D.
                    SIGNATURE

RETURN APPT. ___Post Op_____   DATE _____

OCULAR MOTILITY EXAMINATION

PLATE 13-5

227

Case 5

This 21-year-old patient had an esotropia with a blind spot mechanism. This type of patient is typically resistant to repeated attempts at surgical correction. Only a minimal amblyopia was present. Ductions were limited in a bizarre pattern, as is often the case when repeated surgical procedures have been done. Major amblyoscope testing revealed normal retinal correspondence, but the superimposed images faded in and out and no fusional amplitudes were found. The patient in the primary position measured 26 Δ esotropia near and 28 Δ esotropia distance without glasses. A minimal A pattern was present.

Such a patient who has failed to respond to previous surgery will very likely fail to do so again. However, if surgery is decided upon, because of the patient's desire and his unacceptable appearance, my choice would be to do a double 80% marginal myotomy of one medial rectus and a resection of approximately 5.0 mm of one lateral rectus. The eye chosen would depend upon forced ductions done at the time of surgery. A bare sclera closure would be done over the medial rectus since scarring from previous surgery would reduce the weakening effect of the myotomy.

It is very important to explain to the family that anything from no correction to a large overcorrection could be obtained from such surgery. The surgeon must be realistically discouraging.

AGE ONSET	HX:ET all of life, surgery x 4 but still ET, good health, neg. fam. HX, occasional diplopia	AGE NOW
? Birth		21 yrs.

GLASSES (/ /)	OCCLUSION	ORTHOPTICS	SURGERY
OD +.50	OD age 3 for		1) Bimed. recession
OS +.25	6 mos.	NO	2) Bilat. LR resection
ADD			3) Recess MR OD
			4) Recess MR OS
			5) Resect LR OS

VISION	"E" GAME	LINEAR "E"	LETTER CHT.	PIN HOLE	OTHER
				All surgery done elsewhere	
OD	/	/	20/20		
OS	/	/	20/25	/	/

FIXATION	DUCTIONS	SCREEN COMITANCE
Prefers OD, will hold OS	slight limitation of abd and add OU	

HEAD POSTURE   OK

AMBLYOSCOPE	RANGE	SUPP. ± fades in and out
OBJ. = +26	/ TO /	SUPERIMP. Partial
	NO	
SUB. = +26	/ TO /	FUSION 0

STEREO NIL   WORTH OD   BAG.   A.I.

24△ ET

PRISM COVER TEST

DIST. s̄ GL. = 26△ ET OS

DIST. c̄ GL. =

NEAR s̄ GL. = 28△ ET OS

NEAR c̄ GL. =

20△ ET

FIXATION

Cyclogyl Retinoscopy
OD +.50
OS +.25
F: OK

DIAGNOSIS

1) Small angle residual ET with blind spot mechanism.

TREATMENT

Double 80% MM M.R. and reresect L.R. 5.0 mm - Explain possibility of no change or overcorrection.

_____ M.D.
SIGNATURE

RETURN APPT. ____ Post Op ____   DATE _____

PLATE 13-6

Case 6

This patient represented a fairly typical case of sixth nerve palsy. Since this had been present for more than a year, it can be assumed that the maximum regeneration of sixth nerve function had taken place. One should ordinarily wait from 6 to 9 months after an extraocular muscle palsy before considering surgery. In this case, the history indicated completely normal eye function prior to the accident, and this was confirmed by the fact that fusion with amplitudes was obtained on testing with the major amblyoscope. Since abduction of the left eye was limited to the midline, forced duction and active forced generation tests were done. Forced abduction restricted to the midline indicated that adhesions somewhere around the globe and/or spasticity of the medial rectus had supervened. Muscle force generation testing indicated a definite weakness of the left lateral rectus in addition to the mechanical restriction to abduction already noted. The diagnosis of left lateral rectus palsy was further supported by a floating saccade seen on attempted abduction of the left eye.

The surgical treatment indicated in such a case is a muscle transfer procedure. This is so because of the negative muscle force generation test, indicating a weakness of the left lateral rectus. The restriction in forced abduction of the left eye indicates the need also for recession of the medial rectus in addition to the transfer procedure. Because of the need for a medial rectus recession, I would do a Jensen muscle transfer procedure to preserve the nasal anterior ciliary vessels in the superior and inferior rectus muscles. If there had been no restriction to forced abduction, I would do a full tendon transfer, shifting the superior and inferior rectus muscles to a point adjacent to the insertion of the paretic lateral rectus muscles.

If in a case of sixth nerve palsy such as this the forced ductions had been restricted and the active forced generation test had indicated good contractibility of the lateral rectus supported by a saccadic movement of normal velocity in attempted abduction of the left eye, a recession-resection procedure of the horizontal rectus in the left eye would be indicated as a primary procedure.

230

OCULAR MOTILITY EXAMINATION

AGE ONSET	HX: Auto accident 13 mo ago.	AGE NOW
35 yrs	Unconscious 15 min. ET OS present since accident,	36 yrs

nearly constant diplopia worse left gaze, diabetes well controlled, housewife wants help.

GLASSES (/ /)	OCCLUSION	ORTHOPTICS	SURGERY
OD −1.25 +.50 x 90	Alt for 1	NO	NONE
OS −2.00 +.75 x 90	year		
ADD			

VISION	"E" GAME	LINEAR "E"	LETTER CHT	PIN HOLE	OTHER
OD	/	/	20/20	/	J#1
OS	/	/	20/20	/	J#1

FIXATION	DUCTIONS	SCREEN COMITANCE

FIXATION Prefers OD

DUCTIONS Can abduct OS to midline only, forced ductions can abduct OS only few degrees past midline

HEAD POSTURE Left head turn

AMBLYOSCOPE	RANGE	SUPP. NO
OBJ. = +55	∔6 TO −4 /	SUPERIMP. YES
SUB. = +5.5	+20 TO +16	FUSION YES "floating" saccade

STEREO Diplopia WORTH 5   BAG. −   A.I. − A.F. 6 − Weak L.R. contraction

45△ ET

65△ ET

PRISM COVER TEST

DIST. s̄ GL. = 50△ ET OS with OS fixing
                    ET 15△ more
DIST. c̄ GL. = 60△ ET OS

NEAR s̄ GL. = 55△ ET OS

NEAR c̄ GL. = 60△ ET OS

FIXATION

Cyclogyl 1% Retinoscopy
OD
OS   +.25 over present RX

F.D.: 3+ to abduction OS
A.F.G.: Slight pull-weak LR OS
F.: OK

DIAGNOSIS
   1) VI nerve palsy, OS

TREATMENT

   Plan: Jensen Procedure OS, with 3.0 mm recession LMR

_____ M.D.
SIGNATURE

RETURN APPT. ___ Post Op ___   DATE _____

OCULAR MOTILITY EXAMINATION

PLATE 13-7

Case 7

This 5-year-old boy was a rather typical example of intermittent exotropia in childhood. His eyes seemed completely normal except when the left eye "wandered" outward. This, according to the parents, had been occurring with increasing frequency for the preceding 3 years and the exotropia was now apparent nearly half the time.

While no cooperation could be gained on testing with the major amblyoscope, third-degree fusion with good stereopsis and normal retinal correspondence could be determined. Actually, most patients with intermittent exotropia, in spite of having good stereopsis, demonstrate no second-degree fusion on the amblyoscope. The deviation was easy to demonstrate in the distance and measured 35 Δ. However, at near, the deviation was significantly less on initial cover testing. If this pattern had remained, the diagnosis of divergence excess intermittent exotropia would have been made. However, the fact that after prolonged occlusion of one eye the near deviation increased to be nearly equal to the distance deviation indicated that this was a simulated or pseudodivergence excess basic intermittent exotropia. If the deviation were the same distance and near, at initial examination it would be considered a basic exotropia at the onset.

My indications for surgery in intermittent exotropia are fairly conservative. I prefer to follow and observe such patients initially while the family keeps a "report card" of the deviation. Parents are asked to note how often the eye deviates–that is, how many times a day the eye "wanders out"–and also the percentage of the time the eye is out. The progression of intermittent exotropia in such children is usually very slow. Hiles, Davies, and Costenbader pointed out that not all childhood intermittent exotropia is progressive and that some patients actually improve.

When the deviation becomes manifest in the neighborhood of 50% of the time, I feel that surgery is indicated. If surgery can be delayed until age 4 or 5 years, postoperative orthoptics, which may be required in case of an overcorrection, can be more easily employed.

My choice of surgery for basic and simulated divergence excess exotropia is a recession-resection of one eye. In this patient a 6.0-mm lateral rectus recession and 7.0-mm medial rectus resection were indicated. If the patient had a true divergence excess, bilateral 6.0-mm recessions of the lateral rectus would be indicated.

Surgery for intermittent exotropia is done in children if the eyes are exotropic close to 50% of the time. It is done in older patients if the patient is symptomatic or if an adult wants to avoid even occasional periods of manifest exodeviation. The more often and the longer the eyes are deviated, the more likely that surgical intervention is indicated. The amount of surgery in millimeters is indicated by the angle of the deviation. A 30 Δ intermittent requires the same amount of surgery as a 30 Δ constant exotropia.

OCULAR MOTILITY EXAMINATION			

AGE ONSET 2 yrs ?	HX: BW 7#6oz., good health, normal growth and develop-ment, family noted one eye	AGE NOW 5 yrs

wanders out 4 or 5 x's a day at first, now out 50% of time, neg. fam. HX, to start K'garten in 3 mon., child has no eye complaints

---

GLASSES (NONE /) OCCLUSION ORTHOPTICS SURGERY

OD +.75 NO NO NO
OS +.75 Cyclo 1% Retinos-
  ADD copy

VISION	"E" GAME	LINEAR "E"	LETTER CHT.	PIN HOLE	OTHER
OD	/	20/ 30	/	/	/
OS	/	20/ 30	/	/	/

FIXATION DUCTIONS SCREEN COMITANCE

Fusion to OS out OK

HEAD POSTURE OK NPC - to nose

AMBLYOSCOPE RANGE SUPP.

OBJ. = / TO / SUPERIMP.
  NO COOP
SUB. = / TO / FUSION

STEREO "C" 6/9 WORTH 4D N BAG. X A.I.

36Δ X(T) PRISM COVER TEST

DIST. $\bar{s}$ GL. = 35Δ X(T) fair recovery

DIST. $\bar{c}$ GL. =

NEAR $\bar{s}$ GL. = 15Δ X(T) mostly X

30Δ X(T) NEAR $\bar{c}$ GL. = occlusion for 2 hours brings
  near deviation to 32Δ X(T) F: OK

FIXATION

DIAGNOSIS

1) Intermittent exotropia, simulated divergence excess

TREATMENT

Recess L.R. OS 6.0 mm, Resect M.R. OS 7.0 mm

_____ M.D.
SIGNATURE

RETURN APPT. _____ Post Op _____ DATE _____

OCULAR MOTILITY EXAMINATION	

PLATE 13-8

Case 8

This adult had a large angle sensory exotropia of the right eye and wanted cosmetic surgery for understandable reasons. The extent of this deviation was more than can ordinarily be eliminated with a recession-resection procedure done on one eye, but the patient had some reservations about having her good, left eye operated on. This was also understandable; but, in order to correct this large deviation, more than the usual amount of surgery would be required on the right eye.

In this patient I would do an 8.0-mm right lateral rectus recession, a large (up to 14.0-mm) right medial rectus resection, and, at the same procedure, an 80% double marginal myotomy of the already recessed lateral rectus muscle. This produces a double weakening effect on the lateral rectus while allowing this muscle to retain a reasonable physiologic arc of contact.

In general, patients who have very poor vision in one eye and who want cosmetic surgery are hesitant to have the sound eye operated. In spite of the fact that the morbidity of extraocular muscle surgery is extremely low, this does seem like a reasonable attitude on the part of the patient. In such cases I attempt to accomplish the surgical goals by working only on the poorer eye. This, however, does not apply in every case. As has been pointed out by Knapp, it is occasionally advisable to operate on the fixing eye in certain cases with amblyopia. If compelling reasons are present, operation on the sound eye certainly can and should be done.

These case reports serve as an example of the general thought processes that should be carried out each time that strabismus surgery is contemplated. This type of preplanning holds obvious benefits for the patient. In addition, with this type of planning, the surgeon has a better opportunity to know why a certain procedure succeeded and, on the other hand, why a procedure may have failed.

OCULAR MOTILITY EXAMINATION

AGE ONSET 6 yrs.	HX: XT since early childhood, poor vision in right eye, was told nothing could be	AGE NOW 51 yrs.

done for vision or XT, health good wants cosmetic surgery.

GLASSES (/ /)	OCCLUSION	ORTHOPTICS	SURGERY
OD + .75 +.50 x 100	NO	NO	NO
OS +1.00 +.25 x 90			
ADD +1.50			

VISION	"E" GAME	LINEAR "E"	LETTER CHT.	PIN HOLE	OTHER
OD	/	/	20/300	/	J#10
OS	/	/	20/20	/	J#1

FIXATION	DUCTIONS	SCREEN COMITANCE
OS	Limited adduction	
	Excess abduction OD	

HEAD POSTURE OK   NPC - Remote

AMBLYOSCOPE	RANGE	SUPP.
OBJ. =	/ TO /	SUPERIMP.
SUB. = Unable	/ TO /	FUSION

STEREO NIL   WORTH OS   BAG.   A.I. -   Toxo lesion

PRISM COVER TEST

DIST. s̄ GL. =

DIST. c̄ GL. =   75Δ XT   OD Krimsky

NEAR s̄ GL. =

NEAR c̄ GL. =   80Δ XT   OD Krimsky

FIXATION

F: OK - OS

DIAGNOSIS

1) Sensory Exotropia

TREATMENT

1) Recess RLR 8.0 mm
2) Resect RMR 10.0+ up to 14.0 mm
3) 80% double marginal myotomy of RLR

_____ M.D.
SIGNATURE

RETURN APPT. ___ Post Op ___   DATE _____

OCULAR MOTILITY EXAMINATION

PLATE 13-9

DIAGNOSIS OF ISOLATED CYCLOVERTICAL MUSCLE PALSY
Two step test

Diagnosis of an isolated cyclovertical muscle palsy may be accomplished with a simple two step test.* The two step test is done as follows:

Step 1. The patient, while seated facing the examiner, is asked to look to his right and then to his left. Cover testing or simple observation is used to determine in which lateral gaze the vertical deviation is greater. While in the lateroversion of greater vertical tropia the adducted eye will be either hyperdeviated or hypodeviated. This vertically deviated eye while in adduction "looks at" the *pair* of possibly paretic muscles. This pair includes the *oblique* on the same side as the adducted eye and the *rectus* on the opposite side. This pair of muscles is either *superior* or *inferior*. Step 1 actually combines steps 1 and 2 of Park's three step test.

Step 2. The patient's head is tilted first to his right shoulder and then to his left shoulder. If the vertical deviation increases while the head is tilted toward the side of the higher eye, the *oblique* muscle from the pair implicated in step 1 is paretic. If the vertical deviation is greater while the head is tilted toward the side of the lower eye, the *rectus* muscle implicated in step 1 is parectic.

PLATE 13-10

This case demonstrates a patient in whom the two step test was positive for a right superior oblique palsy.

A In the lateroversion of greater vertical tropia, the adducted eye "looks at" the right superior oblique and the left superior rectus as the possibly paretic muscles.

B The head tilt test indicates that the vertical tropia is greater when the head is tilted toward the higher eye, implicating the oblique from step 1. The diagnosis was right superior oblique palsy.

---

*In complicated cases of vertical strabismus, prism and cover testing in the primary position and the diagnostic positions as well as testing of diplopia fields with a red lens over one eye and the double Maddox rod testing may be required to arrive at the proper diagnosis.

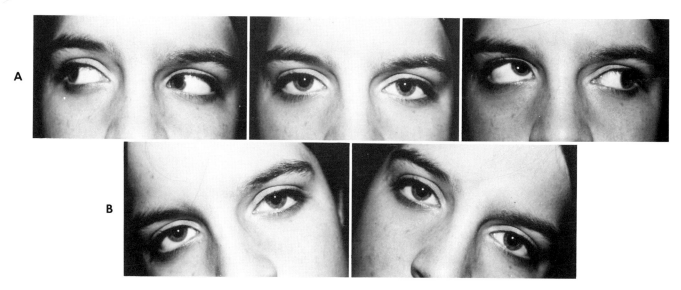

PLATE 13-10

237

SUPERIOR OBLIQUE PALSY

The most common vertical muscle palsy occurring in all ages affects the superior oblique muscle. In children this is usually either congenital or traumatic. In adults, superior oblique palsy may be caused by a late-appearing congenital weakness, trauma, vascular disease, diabetes, or tumor.

When diagnosis of a superior oblique palsy is made, the extent to which the patient should be "worked up" varies and therefore must be individualized. In children with an obvious congenital superior oblique palsy, no special investigation need be carried out. If a congenital etiology is not likely, children as well as adults require examination by an internist and/or neurologist who may request x-rays of the skull, a gulcose tolerance test, a brain scan, cerbral arteriography, or other tests. Such tests should be done only when justified and with the full awareness that these tests are expensive, sometimes dangerous, and usually shed very little light in most cases of isolated superior oblique palsy. The workup therefore should be carried out with discretion.

Knapp proposed a useful scheme for the surgical treatment of superior oblique palsy in all of its manifestations. Seven categories of superior oblique palsy are included in this classification and are divided according to the pattern of the concomitance. Specific muscles are then operated upon to eliminate this concomitance.

PLATE 13-11

A *Class I:* Deviation is greatest in the field of action of the antagonist (inferior oblique).
Treatment: Inferior oblique weakening.

B *Class II:* Deviation is greatest in the field of action of the paretic superior oblique.
Treatment: Superior oblique tuck.

C *Class III:* Deviation is greatest in the entire "opposite" field.
Treatment: For a deviation less than 25 Δ, superior oblique tuck. For a deviation greater than 25 Δ, superior oblique tuck combined with inferior oblique weakening.

D *Class IV:* Deviation is the same in the entire "opposite" field and in down gaze (L shaped pattern).
Treatment: (1) Superior oblique tuck and inferior oblique myectomy; (2) resection of ipsilateral inferior rectus later if necessary.

E *Class V:* Deviation is present "across the bottom" primarily in down gaze and simulating a double elevator palsy or double depressor palsy, depending on which eye is fixating.
Treatment: Tuck in ipsilateral superior oblique, tenectomy of contralateral superior oblique.*

---

*In this last category a recession-resection of the contralateral vertical rectus muscles may be done if the ductions are normal in the involved eye.

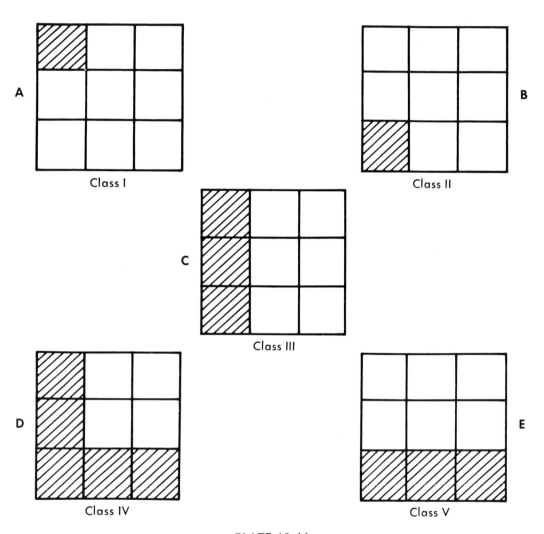

A   Class I

B   Class II

C   Class III

D   Class IV

E   Class V

PLATE 13-11

SUPERIOR OBLIQUE PALSY—cont'd

Class VI: Bilateral superior oblique palsy produces a typical clinical picture. It is treated with a bilateral superior oblique tuck, which is my preference, or by doing a bilateral inferior oblique myectomy. A torsional strabismus greater than 15° is highly indicative of bilateral superior oblique palsy. These patients usually put their chin down and look upward in attempts to fuse.

Class VI   1. Underaction SO, OU
                2. Overaction IO, OU
                3. V pattern
                4. Excyclotropia
                5. Bilaterally positive Bielschowsky test

PLATE 13-12

Class VII: The "canine tooth syndrome" (which incidentally was caused by a dog bite in the patient illustrated) should be treated if significant strabismus is present in the primary position or if the patient is symptomatic. Neither of these was present in this patient. Freeing of restrictions in the trochlear area will improve elevation, and weakening of the yoke (contralateral inferior rectus) will improve the deviation in the down gaze. The canine tooth syndrome in this case shows limited elevation in adduction in the left eye. The scar was produced by a dog's bite. The trochlea was apparently damaged by the bite.

Class VII   The canine tooth syndrome. Underaction inferior oblique (acquired Brown's), underaction superior oblique. Usually caused by trauma in the area of the trochlea

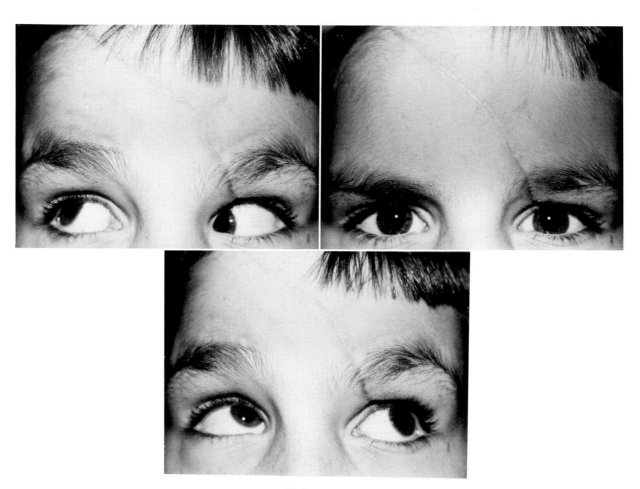

PLATE 13-12

NYSTAGMUS

Nystagmus surgery is indicated in certain patients who assume a cosmetically objectionable head turn in order to place their eyes in the gaze that achieves their nystagmus null point and therefore enables better vision. My choice of surgery for nystagmus is the "straight flush" approach. This technique was suggested by Parks as a modification of previous nystagmus surgery techniques. Muscle procedures of 5.0, 6.0, 7.0, and 8.0 mm are done. This will ordinarily treat 25° of head turn. For more head turn larger numbers may be used. The usual "numbers" are divided so that the amount of surgery in millimeters equals 13 in each eye. The larger numbers are associated with resections and with the lateral rectus, the smaller numbers with the medial rectus and recessions. The surgical procedure is designed so that the same effort is expended postoperatively to keep the yes in the primary position as was needed preoperatively to keep the eyes in the lateroversion associated with the null point of the nystagmus. Therefore the null point of nystagmus is shifted to or nearly to straight-ahead gaze. This "straight flush" procedure enables the patient to retain whatever fusion was present preoperatively.

PLATE 13-13

A "Straight flush" 5, 6, 7, 8. The numbers are divided so that a total of 13.0 mm of surgery is done in each eye.

B The patient preoperatively turns his head to the left (right gaze null point) to obtain better vision. To improve this head posture the eyes must be shifted to the left, in the direction of the head turn. The same neurologic input will then be required postoperatively to place the eyes at or near the primary, or straight-ahead, position as was required to put the eyes in right gaze preoperatively. By this surgery the null point of nystagmus is shifted from right gaze to the primary position.

$$\left.\begin{array}{l}\text{The right lateral rectus is recessed 6.0 mm}\\\text{The right medial rectus is resected 7.0 mm}\end{array}\right\} = 13.0 \text{ mm}$$

$$\left.\begin{array}{l}\text{The left medial rectus is recessed 5.0 mm}\\\text{The left lateral rectus is resected 8.0 mm}\end{array}\right\} = 13.0 \text{ mm}$$

When head turns from nystagmus and strabismus coexist a recession-resection is done on the fixing eye, shifting this eye in the direction of the head turn. A recession-resection is then done on the nonfixing eye to reduce the strabismus.

OTHER STRABISMUS ENTITIES REQUIRING SPECIAL SURGICAL TECHNIQUES

Thyroid myopathy can be unilateral or bilateral and usually affects the inferior rectus, causing varying degrees of hypotropia associated with marked restriction of forced elevation. A large recession of the affected inferior rectus utilizing an adjustable suture can enable the eyes to return to the primary position in most cases. The recession may be as large as 10.0 or 15.0 mm in certain cases. However, such a large recession should be done only after complete dissection of any

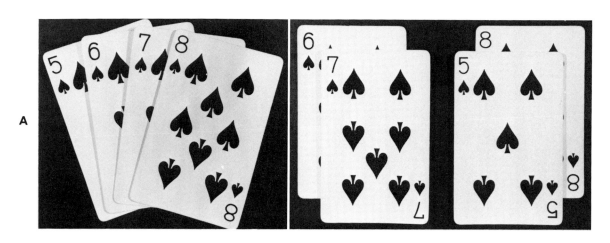

A

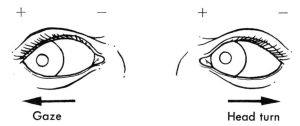

Preoperative

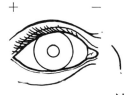

Gaze

Null point in dextroversion

Head turn

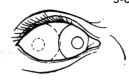

Surgery
"Straight flush"
5-6-7-8

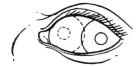

13 mm { 6 mm R.L.R. recession
{ 7 mm R.M.R. resection

13 mm { 5 mm L.M.R. recession
{ 8 mm L.L.R. resection

B

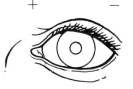

Null point
straight ahead*
No head turn

*Same effort
expended as in
preoperative
dextroversion

PLATE 13-13

243

adhesions that unite the inferior rectus and surrounding structures such as the globe, Lockwood's ligament, inferior oblique, and so on. As might be expected, a certain degree of ptosis of the lower lid results, but this is a small price to pay in light of the marked improvement in motility that usually follows inferior rectus recession.

Möbius syndrome is the result of congenital bilateral sixth nerve and seventh nerve palsy. It causes a marked esotropia with restricted forced abduction as well as absence of nasolabial folds, drooling, an expressionless face, and weakness of the tongue. The ocular alignment may be improved with a large recession of both medial rectus muscles and a large resection of both lateral rectus muscles.

A *blow-out fracture* of the floor or medial wall of the orbit may cause limitation of motility because of acute muscle or fascial entrapment, soft tissue adhesions developing days to weeks after the injury, or the surgical repair of the fracture itself. The last may be caused by muscle impingement by a large plate used in repair of the floor defect. These mechanical restrictions in motility must be freed with careful dissection (and sometimes removal of the plate if previous surgery has been done) until forced or passive ductions are unrestricted on the operating table. Appropriate recession or resection of the extraocular muscles, conjunctival recession, Supramid sheet implants, and traction sutures are then employed. The type of surgery depends on the direction and magnitude of the deviation as well as on the findings after testing passive ductions. Unless forced ductions are free at the time of operation, little hope can be held for significantly improved motility.

Duane's syndrome is characterized by esotropia, limited abduction, enophthalmos with narrowing of the palpebral fissures on attempted adduction, and overaction of the superior or inferior oblique in adduction. Duane's syndrome may be caused by either congenital fibrosis of the lateral rectus or co-contraction of the horizontal recti. Treatment is usually withheld unless a cosmetically objectionable esotropia is present in the primary position or a significant head turn is assumed to enable fusion. When surgery is indicated it usually consists of a large recession of the medial rectus only or a Jensen muscle transfer procedure.

Brown's superior oblique tendon sheath syndrome is characterized by an inability to elevate the eye in adduction. This condition is usually congenital but may be acquired. Surgical treatment should only be attempted if the vertical deviation in the primary position produces a cosmetic defect or if a cosmetically objectionable head position is assumed. Surgery consists of freeing any restrictions associated with the tendon between the trochlea and the medial border of the superior rectus. This dissection should be carried out until forced elevation in adduction is free. The eye may then be fixed in elevation and adduction with a traction suture brought out through the brow nasally. This traction suture is left in place from 5 to 7 days. In rare cases, the restriction of elevation may be associated with abnormal fibrous bands in the inferior temporal quadrant. If dissection around the superior oblique tendon does not lead to improved forced elevation in adduction, the surgeon should then explore the inferior temporal quadrant. Fibrous bands associated with the inferior oblique and with the lateral rectus have been shown to cause a Brown's-like syndrome. Removal of these adhesive bands can lead to

244

a marked improvement in ocular motility. Since dissection around the superior oblique tendon rarely results in a freeing of elevation in adduction, in many cases I have performed a tenectomy of the superior oblique tendon. Crawford has reported good results with this procedure. However, underaction of the superior oblique and a hypertropia in the involved eye can occur. I prefer to operate on Brown's syndrome only if symptoms or appearance indicate a definite need for surgery.

Orbital fibrosis syndrome is characterized by bilateral ptosis, bilateral hypotropia, spasms of convergence on attempted up gaze resulting in an A pattern and limited forced elevation and forced abduction in the midline and above. This condition is inherited as an autosomal dominant trait, and it is not unusual to see three or more members of a family in two generations at the same visit. The surgical treatment of this condition in our hands has consisted of recession of both the medial and inferior rectus and bilateral ptosis surgery consisting of a suture–reinforced, scleral sling brow suspension. At the time of surgery the medial rectus appears to be coursing anteriorly from an origin well below the usual. In spite of vigorous surgical efforts, our experience has been that most patients who have severe involvement derive only a moderate benefit from surgery.

Myasthenia gravis and progressive external ophthalmoplegia often cause severe, incomitant paretic and restrictive strabismus. Attempts at functional cure with surgery are uniformly unsuccessful. Occasionally, surgery on the extraocular muscles is done for cosmetic reasons provided the patient can cope with the inevitable diplopia.

Dissociated vertical deviation, occurring alone or with horizontal or vertical strabismus, is being treated surgically more often than in the past. The general aim of surgery for cosmetically unacceptable dissociated vertical deviation is to weaken the elevators or strengthen the depressors of the eye, either unilaterally or bilaterally. Included among the surgical options are superior rectus recession, inferior oblique weakening, inferior rectus resection, and superior rectus posterior fixation suture (Faden operation). The latter operation is designed to weaken the superior rectus in its field of action while leaving it unaffected in the primary position or in the field of action of the antagonist. Superior oblique "strengthening" to my knowledge has not been suggested as a surgical option for dissociated vertical deviation.

Bibliography

Apt, L., and others: Cat gut allergy in eye muscle surgery, Arch. Ophthalmol. **65:**474-480, 1961.

Berke, R. N.: Tenotomy of the superior oblique for hypertropia, Trans. Am. Ophthalmol. Soc. **44:**304-342, 1946.

Biesner, D. H.: Extraocular muscle recession utilizing silicone tendon prosthesis, Arch. Ophthalmol. **83:**195-204, 1970.

Breinin, G. M.: Accommodative strabismus and the AC/A ratio, Am. J. Ophthalmol. **71:**303-311, 1971.

Brown, H. W.: Congenital structural muscle anomalies. In Allen, J. H., editor: Strabismus ophthalmic symposium I, St. Louis, 1950, The C. V. Mosby Co., pp. 205-236.

Brueggemann, W. G., and Helveston, E. M.: Ketamine anesthesia, Ophthalmic. Surg. **2(6):**243-245, 1971.

Burian, H. M.: Normal and anomalous correspondence. In Allen, J. H., editor: Strabismus ophthalmic symposium II, St. Louis, 1958, The C. V. Mosby Co.

Burian, H. M.: Exodeviations: their classification, diagnosis, and treatment, Am. J. Ophthalmol. **62:**1161-1166, 1966.

Burian, H. M., and von Noorden, G. K.: Binocular vision and ocular motility, St. Louis, 1974, The C. V. Mosby Co.

Chamberlain, W.: The single medial rectus recession operation, J. Pediatr. Ophthalmol. **7(4):**208-211, 1970.

Cooper, E. L.: The surgical management of secondary exotropia, Trans. Am. Acad. Ophthalmol. Otolaryngol. **65:**595-608, 1961.

Crawford, J. S.: Surgical treatment of true Brown's syndrome, Am. J. Ophthalmol. **81(3),** March, 1976.

Crone, R. A.: Diplopia, Amsterdam, 1973, Excerpta Medica.

Dunlap, E. A.: Plastic implants in muscle surgery, Trans. Am. Ophthalmol. Soc. **65:**393-470, 1967.

Dunlap, E. A.: Survey of sutures used in strabismus surgery, Am. J. Ophthalmol. **74(4):**625-626, 1972.

Dunlap, E. A., and others: New uses of ocular adhesives, Arch. Ophthalmol. **82:**756-760, 1969.

Dyer, J. A.: Tenotomy of the inferior oblique muscle at its scleral insertion, Arch. Ophthalmol. **68:**176-181, 1962.

Ellis, F. D., and Helveston, E. M., editors: Strabismus surgery international ophthalmology clinics, Boston, Fall, 1976, Little, Brown and Co., vol. 16, no. 3.

Emery, J. M., von Noorden, G. K., and Schlernitzour, D. A.: Orbital floor fractures: long term follow-up of cases with and without surgical repair, Trans. Am. Acad. Ophthalmol. Otolaryngol. **75:**802, 1971.

Emery, J. M., von Noorden, G. K., and Schlernitzour, D. A.: Management of orbital floor fractures, Am. J. Ophthalmol. **74**(2):299-306, 1972.

Forster, R. C., Paul, O. T., and Jampolsky, A.: Infantile esotropia, Am. J. Ophthalmol. **82**(2):291-299, 1976.

Girard, L. M.: Pseudoparalysis of the inferior oblique muscle, South. Med. J. **49**:342-346, 1956.

Gottlieb, F., and Castro, J. L.: Perforation of the globe during strabismus surgery, Arch. Ophthalmol. **84**:151-157, 1970.

Hardesty, H. H.: Superior oblique tenotomy, Arch. Ophthalmol. **88**(2):181-184, 1972.

Helveston, E. M.: A new disposable headrest for surgery, Am. J. Ophthalmol. **64**(3):468-469, 1967.

Helveston, E. M.: A new two step method for the diagnosis of isolated cyclovertical muscle palsies, Am. J. Ophthalmol. **64**(5):914-915, 1967.

Helveston, E. M.: "A" exotropia, bilateral overaction of the superior obliques and alternating sursumduction, Am. J. Ophthalmol. **67**:377-380, 1969.

Helveston, E. M.: Muscle transposition procedures, Surv. Ophthalmol. **16**(2):92-97, 1972.

Helveston, E. M., Beams, R., Cofield, D. D., and Rohn, R. J.: Strabismus surgery in hemophilia, J. Pediatr. Ophthalmol. **7**:116-117, 1970.

Helveston, E. M., and Callahan, M. A.: Synthetic absorbable suture for strabismus surgery, Am. J. Ophthalmol. **82**(2):1976.

Helveston, E. M., and Cofield, D. D.: Indications for marginal myotomy and technique, Am. J. Ophthalmol. **70**:574-578, 1970.

Helveston, E. M., and Grossman, R. D.: Extraocular muscle lacerations, Am. J. Ophthalmol. **81**(6):300-302, 1976.

Helveston, E. M., and von Noorden, G. K.: Microtropia: a newly defined entity, Arch. Ophthalmol. **78**:272-281, 1967.

Hiles, D. A., Davies, G. T., and Costenbader, F. D.: Long-term observations on unoperated intermittent exotropia, Arch. Ophthalmol. **80**:436-442, 1968.

Jampolsky, A.: Vertical strabismus surgery. In Transactions of the New Orleans Academy of Ophthalmology: Symposium on strabismus, St. Louis, 1971, The C. V. Mosby Co., pp. 366-385.

Jensen, C. D. F.: Rectus muscle union: a new operation for paralysis of the rectus muscles, Trans. Pac. Coast Otoophthalmol. Soc. **45**:359-384, 1964.

Jones, L. T.: A new concept of the orbital fascia and its surgical implications, Trans. Am. Acad. Ophthalmol. Otolaryngol. **72**(5):755-764, 1968.

Knapp, P.: Vertically incomitant horizontal strabismus: the so-called "A" and "V" syndromes, Trans. Am. Ophthol. Soc. **57**:666-699, 1959.

Knapp, P.: The surgical treatment of double-elevator paralysis, Trans. Am. Ophthalmol. Soc. **67**:304-323, 1969.

Knapp, P.: Diagnosis and surgical treatment of hypertropia, Am. Orthopt. J. **21**:29-37, 1971.

Kroczek, S. E., Heyde, E. L., and Helveston, E. M.: Quantifying the marginal myotomy, Am. J. Ophthalmol. **70**:204-209, 1970.

Manley, R. D., and Hughes, R. M.: Surgical management of A pattern esotropia, Ann. Ophthalmol. **3**(10):1067-1078, 1971.

McLean, J. M.: Direct surgery of underacting oblique muscles, Trans. Am. Ophthalmol. Soc. **46**:633-651, 1948.

McLean, J. M., Galin, M. A., and Baras, I.: Retinal perforation during strabismus surgery, Am. J. Ophthalmol. **50**:1167-1169, 1960.

Metz, H. S., and others: Ocular saccades in lateral rectus palsy, Arch. Ophthalmol. **84**:453-460, 1970.

Miller, J. E.: Vertical recti transplantation in the A and V syndromes, Arch. Ophthalmol. **64:**175-179, 1960.

Moore, S.: The prognostic value of lateral gaze measurements in intermittent exotropia, Am. Orthopt. J. **19:**69-71, 1969.

Moore, S., Mein, J., and Stockbridge, L., editors: Orthoptics: past, present, future, Miama, 1976, Symposium Specialists.

Parks, M. M.: Fornix incision for horizontal rectus muscle surgery, Am. J. Ophthalmol. **65**(6):907-915, 1968.

Parks, M. M.: The weakening surgical procedures for eliminating overaction of the inferior oblique muscle, Am. J. Ophthalmol. **73**(1):107-122, 1972.

Parks, M. M.: Ocular motility and strabismus, New York, 1975, Harper & Row, Publishers.

Parks, M. M., and Helveston, E. M.: Direct visualization of the superior oblique tendon, Arch. Ophthalmol. **84:**491-494, 1970.

Pratt-Johnson, J. A.: The surgery of congenital nystagmus, Can. J. Ophthalmol. **6**(4):268-277, 1971.

Reinecke, R. D.: The figure of eight suture for eye muscle surgery, Ophthalmol. Dig. **34:**22-27, 1972.

Romano, P. E., and von Noorden, G. K.: Atypical responses to the four-diopter prism test, Am. J. Ophthalmol. **67:**935-941, 1969.

Scott, A. B.: Active force tests in lateral rectus paralysis, Arch. Ophthalmol. **85:**397-404, 1971.

Scott, A. B., Collins, C. C., and O'Meara, D. M.: A forceps to measure strabismus forces, Arch. Ophthalmol. **88**(3):330-333, 1972.

Scott, A. B., and Knapp, P. K.: Surgical treatment of superior oblique tendon sheath syndrome, Arch. Ophthalmol. **88**(3):282-286, 1972.

Scott, A. B., and Wong, G. Y.: Duane's syndrome, Arch. Ophthalmol. **87**(2):140-147, 1972.

Swan, K. C.: The blind spot mechanism in strabismus. In Allen, J. H., editor: Strabismus ophthalmic symposium II, St. Louis, 1958, The C. V. Mosby Co.

Swan, K. C., and Talbot, T.: Recession under Tenon's capsule, Arch. Ophthalmol. **51:**32-41, 1954.

Urist, M. J.: A lateral version light reflex test, Am. J. Ophthalmol. **63:**808-815, 1967.

Urrets-Zavalia, A., Jr., Solares-Zamora, J., and Olmos, H. R.: Anthropological studies on the nature of cyclovertical squint, Br. J. Ophthalmol. **45:**578-596, 1961.

von Noorden, G. K.: The limbal approach to surgery of the rectus muscles, Arch. Ophthalmol. **80:**94-97, 1968.

von Noorden, G. K.: Modification of the limbal approach to the rectus muscles, Arch. Ophthalmol. **82:**349-350, 1969.

von Noorden, G. K.: Orbital cellulitis following extraocular muscle surgery, Am. J. Ophthalmol. **74**(4):627-629, 1972.

von Noorden, G. K.: Anterior segment ischemia following the Jensen procedure, Arch. Ophthalmol. **94:**845-847, 1976.

von Noorden, G. K.: Nystagmus compensation syndrome, Am. J. Ophthalmol. **82**(2):283-290, 1976.

von Noorden, G. K., and Maumeneee, A. E.: Atlas of strabismus, ed. 3, St. Louis, 1977, The C. V. Mosby Co.

Index

251

259

- 45 yr old c̄ 45 XT (-5.00 myopia OU) c̄ Past H/o XT & R&R OS Did R&R in other eye. ~~after~~ Needs exploration of other eye if you do not know what type of surgery was done —

- 25 yrs old c̄ $\begin{array}{|c|c|}\hline 60 & XT \\\hline 50 & XT \\\hline 30 & XT \\\hline\end{array}$ c̄ I.O. overact bilat.   8 mm Recess LR & off. 8 mm Resect MR   done
  MR moved to apex of V & L.R. to open end of V.

- Past H/o XT in childhood & had bilat. Recess.   Now 18-20 ET (Secondary)